# Beyond Stigma: A Cultural Competency Training for HIV Healthcare Professionals

Crown House Productions

Copyright ©

All Rights Reserved

ISBN 9798877793507

Joseph Santiago

Rebecca Moses

Joseph Crown

Dr. April Goggans

Morris Singletary

Brandon Brown

### Publisher and Author Disclaimer

This book is designed as an educational resource and should be utilized as such. It is crucial to understand that the content provided herein is not meant to replace professional medical advice, diagnosis, or treatment. While every effort has been made to ensure the accuracy and relevance of the information, the authors and the publisher assume no responsibility for any potential adverse effects arising from the application of the concepts and strategies discussed in this book.

As healthcare professionals, you are encouraged to apply your professional judgment and expertise when assimilating and implementing the knowledge presented. It is essential to consider the implications, personal safety aspects, and alignment with your professional and ethical values in your practice. Remember, this book is a tool to enhance your understanding and skills; however, it is not a definitive guide for clinical decision-making. Always prioritize the well-being of your patients and adhere to the latest clinical guidelines and best practices in your field.

This book was created to make your passion projects and dreams come true with the Crown Legacy, Visibility, and Cultural Catalyst Fund. The inspiration for this book originated in the heart of our Giving Circle. As we forge our path, our vision is to evolve into a vibrant community learning network. Our aim extends beyond traditional philanthropy; we are dedicated to discovering and embracing concepts that enable us to leave a lasting, positive imprint on the communities we engage with.

Our approach to giving transcends monetary contributions. We offer a more holistic investment - our time, compassion, intellect, and a diverse array of skills. This multidimensional form of support is designed to forge deeper, more meaningful connections with others. This book is a manifestation of shared experiences and learnings. It aims to share insights on how holistic giving can create ripple effects of positive change. It's a narrative of how a Giving Circle can transform from a group of individual donors into a powerful force for community development and empowerment. Through our journey, we hope to inspire and guide others on how to make the most impact with their giving, creating a network of support that extends far beyond monetary donations.

As you read these words, you are being transported to a place of possibility. A place where your dreams are within reach. A place where you are surrounded by people who believe in you and your vision.

This book is your invitation to join the Crown Legacy, Visibility, and Cultural Catalyst Fund. This fund is dedicated to helping people like you turn their passion projects into reality. We believe that everyone has the potential to make a difference in the world, and we are here to help you make your mark.

As you hold this book in your hands, take a moment to run your fingers across its cover and feel the weight of its pages.

There's an unexplainable energy here that tugs at your senses and ignites your curiosity. You're not just reading a book, you're embarking on a journey of connection with people you've never met. As you earnestly seek, you'll find hidden connections within these passages that continue to resonate with you long after you've put the book down.

It's like having a conversation with a beloved friend who understands your deepest thoughts and desires.

The words on these pages have their own voice and their own energy that speaks to your soul. As you turn each page, you'll feel like you're entering a new world filled with wonder and possibility.

The message within these pages has the power to change minds and inspire action.

It all starts with developing the right energy in each situation and celebrating all that makes you unique. In a world that constantly asks who you are, it's essential to seek silence amidst the noise and listen to where your heart and mind wander. As you hold tight to the harmony within yourself, you'll grow attuned to the world around you and find your true path.

When you're finished reading this book, I invite you to share the messages with others.

Tell your friends, family, and colleagues about the book and what it means to you. Share your thoughts and insights on social media and in online forums. The more people who are exposed to these messages, the more likely they are to make a difference in the world.

Together, we can create a culture of change and transformation.

We can build a world where everyone is celebrated for their unique gifts and talents. We can create a world where everyone has the opportunity to reach their full potential. We can create a world where everyone feels like they belong.

The future is in your hands. What will you do with it?

# Table of Contents

***This work has been brought to you by the Crown Legacy, Visibility, and Cultural Catalyst Fund***

The fund supports and promotes LGBTIQQ, Latino, LatinX, and Hispanic mixed media artists (such as AR, VR, and more!), creators, writers, lifestyle presenters, and culture bearers to create and educate others.

Those underrepresented in the community media and culture will be the focus of the funds as we seek to encourage their voice and the development of passion projects. Everyone can apply, however, a top priority will be given to underserved voices within our communities. Click below if you'd like to donate to this fund and help us with this mission. https://2014givenow.kimbia.com/crownlegacy

Join us in spreading the expression of our world, culture, and passion with open hearts and minds! Help launch and promote the Crown Legacy Visibility and Cultural Catalyst Fund.

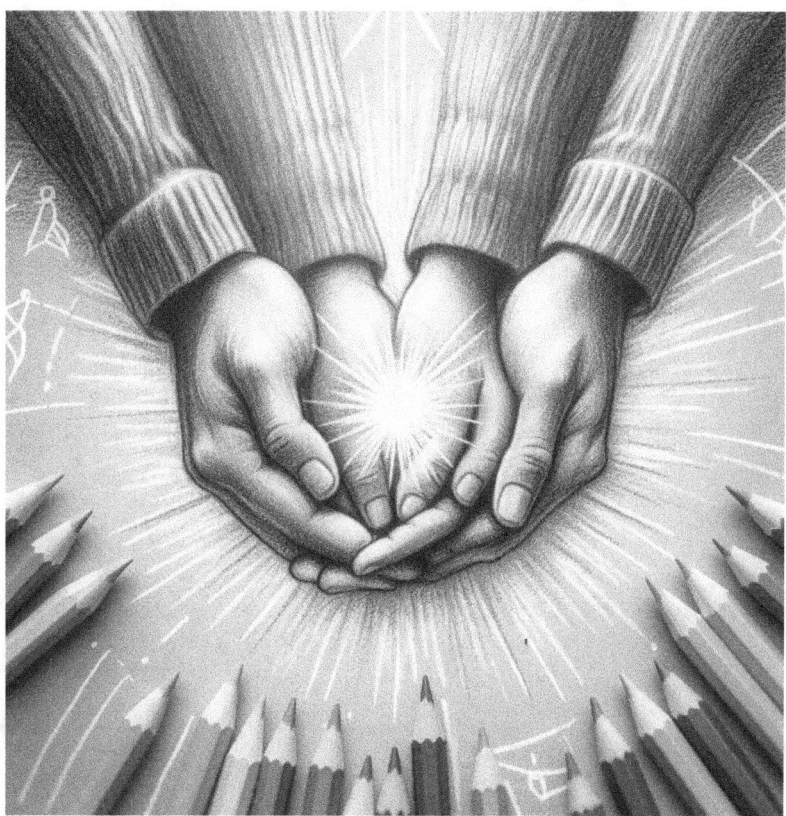

## Dedication

This book is dedicated to the tireless healthcare professionals and community advocates who devote their lives to caring for individuals living with HIV. Your unwavering commitment, compassion, and dedication inspire a world where healthcare is inclusive, empathetic, and free from stigma.

To those who have faced the challenges of HIV, either personally or in supporting a loved one: your strength and resilience light the way towards understanding and hope. May this work honor your journey and contribute to a future where every individual receives the care, respect, and dignity they deserve.

Your authors,

Joseph Santiago

Rebecca Moses

Joseph Crown

Morris Singletary

Brandon Brown

April Goggans

## Foreword

In this captivating prologue to the foreword, we are honored to present the collective voices of distinguished community leaders. Their words embody the spirit of perseverance, unity, and dedication that has shaped the journey towards a more compassionate and inclusive world. These leaders, through their experiences and insights, offer a powerful testament to the resilience and strength found in communities dedicated to supporting individuals living with HIV. As you read their contributions, we invite you to absorb the depth of their wisdom and the shared commitment to a future where healthcare transcends barriers and embraces every individual with dignity and respect. Let their perspectives guide and inspire you on this important journey towards understanding and change.

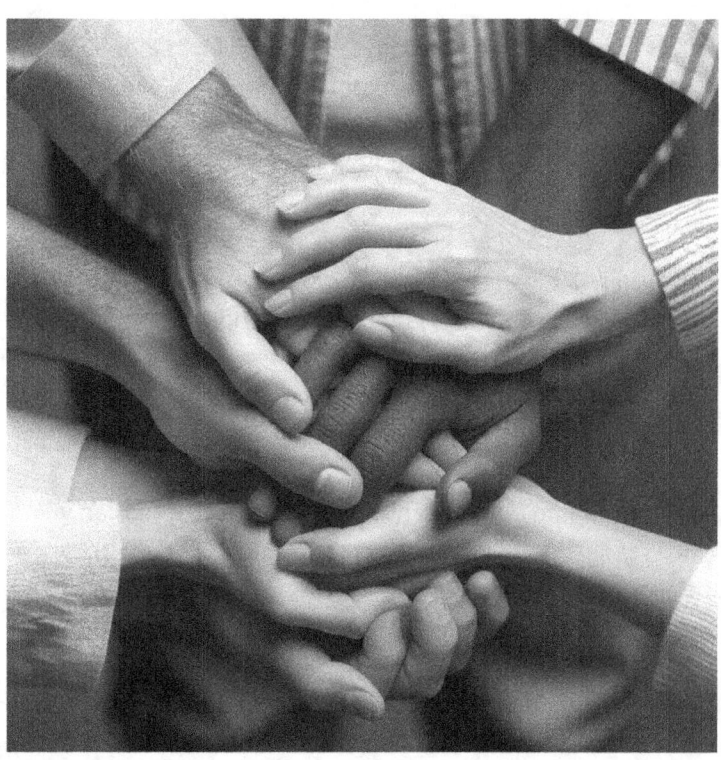

# Foreword by Noel Twilbeck

As I embark on a new chapter in my journey as a Senior Management Specialist at St. Thomas Community Health Center, I am honored to write this foreword and share my insights drawn from years of dedication in the healthcare industry. My experiences, first as the CEO of CrescentCare Health Center and now in my current role, have deeply ingrained in me the importance of understanding, empathy, and continuous learning in healthcare.

This book, centered on building a comprehensive understanding of stigma reduction in healthcare, resonates profoundly with the lessons I've learned and the values I hold dear. Having navigated through various facets of healthcare management, from nonprofit organizations to proposal writing and fundraising, I have witnessed firsthand the transformative power of empathy and informed care in improving patient outcomes.

The unique approach of this book in utilizing narratives instead of traditional role-playing scenarios to address stigma and bias is both innovative and necessary. In my years of experience, I have seen that real change in healthcare practice begins with understanding the stories of those we serve. These narratives are not just stories; they are lived experiences that hold the key to unlocking a more compassionate and effective approach to healthcare.

Throughout my career, especially during my time at CrescentCare Health Center and my academic journey at the University of New Orleans, the significance of empathy in healthcare has been a recurring theme. This book captures that essence by providing a platform for healthcare professionals to reflect, discuss, and understand the multifaceted nature of patient experiences, especially those grappling with stigmatized conditions.

As healthcare providers, we often find ourselves at the intersection of human vulnerability and clinical expertise. This book guides readers on how to navigate this intersection with grace and competence. It encourages us to look beyond our biases and preconceptions, urging us to see our patients as individuals with unique stories and experiences.

In my new role at St. Thomas Community Health Center, I am excited to apply the insights gained from this book and to further my commitment to nurturing an environment where every patient feels heard, understood, and cared for. I encourage each reader to delve into these pages with an open heart and mind, ready to embark on a journey of learning, unlearning, and relearning.

To all my fellow healthcare professionals, let this book be a reminder of the profound impact we can have when we approach our work with empathy, understanding, and a willingness to listen to the stories that shape the lives of those we serve.

With warm regards,

Noel Twilbeck
Senior Management Specialist
St. Thomas Community Health Center

As an Infectious Disease specialist with over a decade of experience in the vibrant city of New Orleans who focuses on the care of people with HIV, I have experienced firsthand the challenges and triumphs in the field of HIV care. My journey began by watching my mother, through her circle of friends and through her volunteer work, lose many friends to AIDS during the 1990s. In her career, she worked on research studies in HIV, including some of the early HIV vaccine trials. Her dedication to and passion for people with HIV inspired me, I began my journey into the field of HIV with a medical degree from Thomas Jefferson University. Following Hurricane Katrina, I moved to New Orleans for my residency and fellowship and fell in love with the city and the talented and compassionate people working in the field of HIV. The enduring resilience of people affected by this disease amazed me then and continues to amaze me. I am grateful each day for the opportunity to be part of their lives in such an intimate way, as their physician.

In this book, we embark on an exploratory journey through the complexities of HIV care, delving into the crucial aspect of stigma reduction and the power of empathy in healthcare. The unique approach of this book, focusing on narratives rather than traditional role-playing, aligns perfectly with the realities of medical practice, where every patient's story is as unique as the treatment they require.

New Orleans, a city known for its rich culture and diversity, has also been a landscape where the HIV epidemic has unfolded in ways that reflect both the challenges and the progress in infectious disease management. At University Medical Center New Orleans, I've seen a myriad of patient experiences, each underscoring the importance of understanding and compassion in medical care. This book encapsulates that very essence, offering healthcare professionals insightful strategies to engage with patients beyond the clinical symptoms and delve into their personal narratives.

As we turn each page, we are reminded that behind every diagnosis is a human story. This book encourages healthcare professionals to listen actively, to understand deeply, and to respond thoughtfully. It's not just about treating a virus; it's about treating a person in their entirety – their hopes, fears, and dreams. The methodologies and insights presented here are more than just theoretical concepts; they are practical tools that I believe can transform the way we approach HIV care. From the healthcare system in New Orleans to society at large, the lessons in this book are applicable and necessary for fostering a stigma-free healthcare environment.

The transformative power of this work lies in its ability to reshape the metaphors by which we live and understand our lives. By adopting a narrative perspective, we gain the ability to reframe our experiences and perceptions, a process crucial for both healthcare professionals and patients alike. This narrative approach empowers us to challenge and change the prevailing metaphors of illness and stigma, replacing them with ones of understanding, empathy, and resilience. It is through these reimagined narratives that we can truly begin to effect change in the healthcare landscape.

I wholeheartedly commend the authors for their unwavering commitment to this vital facet of healthcare. They have crafted a resource that is not only enlightening but also deeply human. This book transcends the traditional boundaries of cultural competency training as it stands as a beacon of hope for a future where stigma no longer hinders access to care, and where every individual's story is not just heard but valued and integrated into their journey of healing and wellness.

Lauren Richey, MD, MPH, FIDSA

Medical Director of the HIV Outpatient Program (HOP)
Professor of Medicine, LSU School of Medicine, New Orleans

New Orleans faces multiple challenges when it comes to addressing its high rates of HIV. To effectively combat this epidemic, interventions must address the virus and the underlying factors contributing to its transmission. This requires a comprehensive approach that addresses issues that New Orleans has some of the highest rates of other sexually transmitted infections, housing instability, illiteracy, poverty, and incarceration. Unfortunately, American politics make it so that there are no incentives to create policies that address systemic racism or poverty, making it difficult for communities to access necessary resources and support, further exacerbating the rates of HIV in cities like New Orleans.

Making matters worse is the stigma and discrimination that accompanies people living with HIV (PLWH). Stigma and discrimination are significant barriers to effective prevention, treatment, care, and support. It affects not only the individuals who are directly stigmatized but also their families, friends, and communities. Again, American politics are to blame for perpetuating stigma and discrimination, especially surrounding HIV. Many advocates and experts agree that Ronald Reagan's hesitation in acknowledging and addressing HIV/AIDS in the 1980s was fueled by stigma and discrimination towards the LGBTQ+ community, who were disproportionately affected by the epidemic, further perpetuating stigma against PLWH.

One of the main ways American politics contributes to stigma is through the rhetoric and language politicians use. In recent years, there has been a rise in divisive and inflammatory language used by political leaders, mainly targeting specific groups of people such as immigrants, religious minorities, and the LGBTQ+ community. This type of language creates an environment of fear and hatred towards these communities, leading to increased discrimination and stigmatization.

Motivated by this incendiary language towards marginalized communities, on World AIDS Day (December 1st), 2014, my wife and I launched 102.3FM WHIV-LP (whivfm.org), a community radio station dedicated to human rights and social justice. I deliberately chose those call letters; it was not an accident. The station is not all about HIV all of the time- there is an HIV-related show, but the point of the call letters was to have show hosts and radio disc jockeys say "WHIV" during the station identification 4 times an hour, 24 hours a day, 7 days a week, 4 weeks a month, 12 months a year and now we are approaching 10 years- a decade—a decade of having the word "WHIV" being said over and over again on the New Orleans airwaves.

Words hold immense power. They can either uplift or harm individuals, communities, and societies. As a society, we have associated HIV with fear, shame, and stigma for decades. However, by naming the radio station WHIV, we can use language to change perceptions and break down barriers. By repeatedly using the word "WHIV" on air, we reclaim its negative connotations and turn it into a symbol of empowerment and solidarity.

In New Orleans, we have a local tradition of dropping the 'W" when talking about radio stations. For example, WTUL is known locally as T-U-L. WWOZ, with its two 'W's,' is known as O-Z. And WHIV? The 'W' is dropped, and now, when someone approaches me to talk about HIV, it takes me a moment to determine if they are referring to the virus or the radio station. That's how you take power away from a word! We are so proud that WHIV was able to do that.

One of our first shows on WHIV was Proof Positive, hosted by Dorian-Gray Alexander. Dorian, a gay black male, is a person living with HIV- and a stutter, in the American deep South. Dorian hosted a magnificent show on living with HIV. Through his show, Dorian advocated for those living with HIV. He promoted acceptance and love for all individuals, regardless of their HIV status. His positive outlook and determination to fight against stigma serve as an inspiration to many.

Not long after WHIV went on air, the World Health Organization recruited me to Sierra Leone to fight the Ebola crisis in Freetown- the outbreak's epicenter. After my arrival, I met with representatives from UNAIDS. In casual conversation, I mentioned having just started WHIV and spoke about the Proof Positive show. They asked if I could provide recordings of the show, which I did. They took those recordings and played them in the waiting rooms of UNAIDS HIV clinics.

In many parts of the world, including West Africa, there is still a lot of stigma and discrimination surrounding HIV, leading to individuals living with HIV feeling isolated, ashamed, and afraid to seek treatment or even disclose their status to others. However, having someone like Dorian share his stories and experiences can help break down these barriers and show that living with HIV is not something to be ashamed of.

Representation matters, especially when it comes to marginalized communities such as individuals living with HIV. Listening to someone like Dorian, who is openly living with HIV and thriving, can be incredibly empowering for others who are also going through similar experiences. Proof Positive was a show on WHIV that we were so proud of as it undisputedly fought stigma in New Orleans and West Africa!

During the COVID epidemic, I was fortunate to receive funding to make animations about public health topics such as the COVID mRNA vaccines, hepatitis C, and HIV; you can find all of the animations at noisefiltershow.com. When we looked at making animations about HIV, we decided that we wanted to explain U=U (undetectable equals Untransmittable), PrEP, and nPEP (HIV prevention). As an infectious diseases physician, those topics are near and dear to my heart, and I lecture on them regularly. Beyond using the animations as tools to explain these innovative HIV topics, we decided to use these animations as stigma-fighting weapons. So, who is the perfect person who can be animated and help fight HIV stigma? New Orleans local Milan Nicole Sherry. Milan is a person of trans experience; she is an activist and a person who is living with HIV. She was the perfect stigma-fighting weapon and did it with high heels.

In our animated series, we purposefully featured Milan Nicole Sherry, a person of trans experience living with HIV, as the central character. Milan, along with Doc Griggs (my animation partner) and myself, navigated the complexities of HIV education. This deliberate choice was aimed at bringing to the forefront the experiences of one of the most stigmatized and marginalized groups in society - people of trans experience.

Sadly, individuals in the trans community, particularly Black trans women, frequently face hostility and violence solely based on their gender identity. This harrowing reality, coupled with heightened risks of hate crimes and violence, often forces many into a life shadowed by fear, leading to isolation and increased marginalization. It's imperative that society not only acknowledges but also actively addresses the unique challenges faced by the trans community.

Through our animations, we strive to dismantle the deeply ingrained systems of oppression that perpetuate such stigmatization. By highlighting the stories and perspectives of those like Milan, we aim to foster a greater understanding and acceptance of people of trans experience. Our work is more than just an educational tool; it's a call to action for society to embrace diversity and inclusivity, and to work collectively towards a world where every individual is recognized, respected, and valued for who they are.

In a world where narratives shape our understanding and acceptance, the groundbreaking work of people like Milan Nicole Sherry, Dorian-Gray Alexander, stands as a beacon of change. Their approach, weaving the powerful threads of storytelling with the realities of those living with HIV and trans experiences, is more than educational – it's transformative. They've shown us that through storytelling, we can break down walls of stigma and fear, fostering a world that embraces diversity and nurtures acceptance.

Stories have the power to change the world. They invite us into the lives of others, allowing us to walk in their shoes, feel their joys, and understand their struggles. In a society often divided by differences, storytelling unites us, creating a tapestry of shared human experience. We need more work like this – work that doesn't just tell a story but changes the narrative, one that champions the voices of the marginalized and challenges the status quo.

This book, "Beyond Stigma," is a continuation of this critical mission. It serves as a vital resource for healthcare professionals, echoing the same spirit of storytelling to illuminate the diverse experiences of those affected by HIV. It's more than just a guide; it's a call to action – to listen, to learn, and to transform our perspectives. Through these pages, we extend the work of Milan, Dorian Gray Alexander, and countless others, using narrative-driven approaches to not only educate but also inspire a new generation of empathetic and culturally competent healthcare providers. Together, their work, and this book, pave the way for a more inclusive and understanding world.

Dr. MarkAlain Déry,
Infectious Diseases Physician and Epidemiologist
markalain_dery@hey.com

# Introduction

Welcome to "Beyond Stigma: A Cultural Competency Training for HIV Healthcare Professionals," a comprehensive guide designed to enhance your understanding and skills in caring for individuals living with HIV. This book serves as an essential tool for healthcare professionals and community advocates, focusing on breaking down the barriers of stigma and misinformation surrounding HIV.

Through this training, you will gain a deeper insight into the social determinants of health, understand internalized, external, and associative stigma, and learn the principles of harm reduction and person-first language. The book emphasizes the importance of a narrative-driven approach to build empathy and critical thinking, essential for effective HIV care and stigma reduction.

This book is not just an educational resource; it's a call to action for all healthcare professionals to embrace a more inclusive, understanding, and compassionate approach to HIV care. By engaging with this material, you will be equipped to make a meaningful impact in promoting health equity and improving community well-being.

As you journey through this book, remember that each lesson is a step towards a more empathetic and stigma-free healthcare environment. Your role is crucial in shaping a future where individuals living with HIV receive the care and respect they deserve. Let this book be your guide in making that future a reality.

This book is a workshop that is innovatively designed to accommodate individuals who may find traditional role-playing scenarios challenging or are less experienced in empathetically relating to situations they haven't personally encountered. Unlike role-playing, which requires participants to actively and spontaneously embody characters in simulated situations, this training focuses on sharing and discussing narratives.

Narratives allow participants to engage in a more relaxed setting, encouraging the sharing of stories about their experiences with the people they serve. This method offers a reflective and observational approach, enabling participants to explore various perspectives without the pressure of performance that role-playing often entails.

The narrative approach is particularly effective in addressing implicit biases and fostering empathy. It provides a safe space for healthcare workers to express and examine their preconceptions and attitudes towards stigma. The shared stories act as mirrors, reflecting both personal and collective experiences, allowing biases to surface naturally in a controlled environment.

Conversely, role-playing, while effective in its own right, often places participants directly in the shoes of another, requiring immediate reaction and interaction, which can be daunting for some. It relies heavily on the ability to improvise, empathize, and not hold back or filter in real-time, which might not be conducive for all learning styles, especially for those who are introspective or prefer learning through observation and discussion.

The essence of this training lies in its capacity to challenge behaviors and ideas in a supportive environment, away from the critical eyes of clients. It is an evolving format, continually being refined and tested to maximize its effectiveness in stigma reduction and empathy-building among healthcare professionals. This workshop, therefore, stands as a testament to our commitment to creating inclusive and empathetic healthcare spaces, where narratives serve as powerful tools for learning and personal growth.

We encourage you to actively engage with the exercises, reflect on the case studies, and apply the strategies in your professional practice. By doing so, you'll not only improve your competency but also contribute to a more informed, compassionate healthcare environment. This book is more than a training manual; it's a pathway to change, both in personal practice and in the broader healthcare community. Your participation is vital in shaping a future where stigma is replaced by understanding and quality care for all. Please ensure you follow the steps at the end of this book to get your HIV Stigma Abolitionist (HAS) certification.

This section offers an in-depth exploration of the Social Determinants of Health (SDOH). It is meticulously crafted to enhance the understanding of healthcare professionals, community advocates, and individuals passionate about public health. Grasping the nuances of SDOH is not just an academic exercise; it is a critical element in effectively addressing and reducing health disparities. These determinants play a pivotal role in shaping health outcomes across various populations. By delving into this subject, we aim to equip you with the knowledge and tools necessary to make a meaningful impact in promoting health equity and improving community well-being.

**What are Social Determinants of Health?** Social Determinants of Health (SDOH) refer to the various environmental conditions that significantly influence health outcomes and quality of life. These determinants encompass aspects of where we are born, grow up, live, work, and age. They can be categorized into five key domains, each affecting health and well-being in different ways:

1. **Economic Stability:**

   - **Examples:**

     - Employment: Job security and working conditions can directly impact mental and physical health. For instance, someone with a stable job is likely to have better health outcomes than someone who is unemployed.

     - Income: Higher income levels often provide better access to healthcare services and healthier food options.

     - Expenses and Debt: Financial strain can lead to stress, negatively impacting mental health.

     - Medical Bills: High medical expenses can be a barrier to receiving necessary healthcare.

     - Support: Financial support systems like social welfare can buffer against health crises in economically unstable times.

2. **Education Access and Quality:**

   - **Examples:**

     - Literacy and Language: Being literate and proficient in the dominant language of a region enables better understanding of health information and communication with healthcare providers.

     - Early Childhood Education: High-quality early education sets a foundation for healthy behaviors and knowledge.

     - Vocational Training and Higher Education: Higher levels of education are often linked to better jobs and, consequently, better health coverage and lifestyle.

3. **Healthcare Access and Quality:**

   - **Examples:**

- Health Coverage: Access to health insurance impacts one's ability to receive regular medical care.

- Provider Availability: Having sufficient healthcare providers, especially in rural areas, is crucial for timely and effective medical care.

- Provider Linguistic and Cultural Competency: Healthcare providers who understand a patient's language and culture can offer more personalized and effective care.

- Quality of Care: High-quality healthcare can lead to better disease management and health outcomes.

4. **Neighborhood and Built Environment:**

   - **Examples:**

     - Housing: Living in safe, affordable housing reduces stress and exposure to health hazards.

     - Transportation: Reliable transportation affects the ability to access healthcare, grocery stores, and workplaces.

     - Safety: Neighborhood safety can impact mental health and the ability to engage in outdoor activities.

     - Parks and Playgrounds: Access to recreational areas promotes physical activity and mental well-being.

     - Walkability: Walkable neighborhoods encourage physical activity and community interaction.

5. **Social and Community Context:**

   - **Examples:**

     - Social Integration: Being part of a supportive community can provide emotional support and reduce feelings of isolation.

     - Support Systems: Having a network for social and emotional support can help cope with stress and crises.

     - Community Engagement: Active participation in community events can foster a sense of belonging and collective efficacy.

     - Discrimination: Experiencing discrimination can lead to chronic stress and poor mental health.

     - Stress: Chronic stress, whether from social, economic, or environmental sources, can lead to adverse health effects.

Understanding SDOH is crucial because they can have a profound impact on health outcomes, often more so than genetic or biological factors. Addressing these determinants is key to improving health and reducing longstanding disparities in health and healthcare.

**Why are SDOH Important?** Social Determinants of Health (SDOH) are crucial because they significantly influence health outcomes and disparities. For instance, where a person lives – often captured by their zip code – can have a more telling impact on their health than their genetic makeup. This means a person living in an area with limited access to fresh food and healthcare facilities might have a higher risk of health issues than someone in a more resource-rich neighborhood. Factors like poverty, education quality, and housing stability play pivotal roles in determining health risks and outcomes. For example, living in a poverty-stricken area often correlates with higher rates of illnesses due to inadequate healthcare access, poor nutrition, and stress.

**Strategies for Addressing SDOH:**

**Education and Awareness:**

- **Objective:** Increase public understanding of how SDOH impact health.

- **Example:** Conducting workshops in schools and workplaces to educate people about how lifestyle and environmental factors can affect health. For instance, explaining how living in an area with high air pollution can exacerbate asthma and other respiratory conditions.

**Community Engagement:**

- **Objective:** Work with local organizations to pinpoint and tackle SDOH in specific areas.

- **Example:** Partnering with local food banks and nutritionists to address food deserts (areas lacking in affordable, healthy food options). This collaboration could lead to setting up weekly farmers' markets in these areas, making fresh produce more accessible.

**Policy Advocacy:**

- **Objective:** Promote policies that enhance critical SDOH like housing and healthcare.

- **Example:** Lobbying for legislation that provides funding for affordable housing projects, ensuring that more people have access to safe and stable living conditions, which is fundamental to maintaining good health.

**Integrated Healthcare Services:**

- **Objective:** Develop healthcare models that incorporate social needs along with medical treatment.

- **Example:** A clinic that not only offers medical care but also has on-site social workers who can assist patients with finding housing, job training, or mental health services. Such an integrated approach ensures a more holistic care system, addressing both the medical and social needs of patients.

By understanding and addressing SDOH effectively, it's possible to create healthier communities and reduce health disparities, leading to an overall improvement in public health. Understanding and effectively addressing Social Determinants of Health (SDOH) is crucial in fostering healthier communities and reducing health disparities. This leads to a significant improvement in public health overall.

For example, consider access to nutritious food, a key SDOH. In areas with limited access to fresh produce (often called "food deserts"), residents might rely more on processed foods, leading to higher rates of obesity and related health issues. By improving access to healthy food options, perhaps through community gardens or subsidized grocery stores, these health risks can be mitigated.

Another SDOH is the availability of safe, affordable housing. Living in overcrowded or unsafe conditions can lead to chronic stress, exposure to environmental hazards, and increased spread of infectious diseases. Initiatives like affordable housing projects or improved housing regulations can directly impact the physical and mental well-being of community members.

Education is also a significant determinant. Higher levels of education often correlate with better health outcomes. By investing in quality education and making it accessible to all, communities can empower individuals with knowledge about health practices, leading to healthier lifestyles.

Employment and working conditions also play a role. Job security and safe, fair work environments contribute to reduced stress and better mental health. Efforts to ensure fair wages and safe working conditions can thus improve overall community health.

In essence, by targeting these and other SDOH, communities can tackle the root causes of health disparities. This not only improves the well-being of individuals but also contributes to a healthier, more equitable society as a whole.

## Knowledge Check

Welcome to the Knowledge Check sections! These segments are designed to enhance your understanding and retention of key concepts discussed in our training. Each section presents a series of thought-provoking questions or problems that will challenge your grasp of the material. By engaging with these questions, you'll have the opportunity to reflect on what you've learned, apply your knowledge in practical scenarios, and deepen your comprehension of the subject matter. These checks are a vital part of the learning process, enabling you to consolidate your learning and identify areas where you may need further clarification or study. Let's dive in and explore these concepts further!

1. **Question:** How does limited access to healthcare impact the management and prevention of HIV in a community?

**Answer:** Limited access to healthcare significantly impedes effective management and prevention of HIV. People living in areas with inadequate healthcare services may face delays in HIV testing and diagnosis, leading to late initiation of antiretroviral therapy (ART). For example, in rural areas without nearby clinics, individuals might not get tested for HIV until symptoms become severe. Early detection and timely treatment are crucial for managing HIV effectively, as they reduce the viral load, improve health outcomes, and decrease the risk of transmission. Furthermore, without regular access to healthcare, individuals with HIV may struggle to adhere to ART regimens, leading to poorer health outcomes and increased community viral load.

2. **Question:** Explain how stigma and discrimination related to HIV status can affect an individual's mental health and access to treatment.

**Answer:** Stigma and discrimination can have profound effects on the mental health of individuals living with HIV. They may experience social isolation, depression, and anxiety due to fear of judgment or rejection from their community. This stigma not only impacts their mental well-being but can also deter them from seeking treatment. For instance, an individual might avoid going to a clinic for HIV care due to fear of being seen and stigmatized. This can lead to delayed treatment, which can worsen health outcomes. Additionally, internalized stigma – where the individual adopts these negative beliefs about themselves – can lead to a lack of self-care and adherence to treatment. It's essential to combat HIV-related stigma to ensure individuals feel safe and supported in accessing and adhering to their treatment.

3. **Question:** How do socioeconomic factors influence the risk of HIV transmission in certain populations?

**Answer:** Socioeconomic factors play a significant role in influencing the risk of HIV transmission. People in lower socioeconomic groups often have limited access to education, including sexual health education, leading to a lack of awareness about HIV prevention methods such as condoms and pre-exposure prophylaxis (PrEP). For example, young people from underprivileged backgrounds might not receive comprehensive sex education, increasing their risk of HIV. Additionally, economic constraints can lead to increased vulnerability, such as engaging in transactional sex for financial support, further elevating the risk of HIV transmission. Addressing these socioeconomic disparities is crucial in reducing the risk of HIV transmission.

4. **Question:** Discuss the role of housing instability in the health outcomes of people living with HIV.

**Answer:** Housing instability significantly impacts the health outcomes of individuals living with HIV. Stable housing is a crucial factor for effective management of HIV, as it influences the ability to store medication properly, maintain a consistent treatment regimen, and attend regular medical appointments. People experiencing housing instability or homelessness may find it challenging to adhere to their ART regimen, leading to poorer health outcomes and higher viral loads. For instance, someone without a stable place to live might miss doses of their medication or lose access to their healthcare provider, hindering their ability to manage their HIV effectively. Ensuring stable housing is therefore a key component in supporting the health and well-being of people living with HIV.

These questions and answers are designed to test and improve understanding of the complex interplay between Social Determinants of Health and HIV, emphasizing the importance of addressing these determinants to improve health outcomes for people living with HIV.

This training document serves as a resource to understand and address internalized HIV stigma. It aims to provide healthcare professionals, community advocates, and individuals with essential knowledge and strategies to combat the internalization of HIV-related stigma.

## What is Internalized HIV Stigma?

**Definition:** Internalized stigma is the personal acceptance of prejudice and discrimination based on an HIV-positive status. It's when individuals believe the negative stereotypes and societal judgments about HIV apply to themselves.

- **Examples of Manifestations:**

  - **Shame:** Feeling embarrassed about one's status, like a young man who avoids social gatherings for fear his HIV status might be revealed.

  - **Self-Blame:** Blaming oneself for their condition, such as a woman believing she 'deserves' her diagnosis due to past choices.

  - **Fear of Disclosure:** Worrying about others' reactions, exemplified by someone who hides their medication to prevent questions from friends or family.

  - **Sense of Worthlessness:** Believing one is no longer valuable, seen in individuals who withdraw from relationships and community involvement.

- **Impact on Individuals:** Internalized stigma can sabotage mental health, leading to depression or anxiety, and deter individuals from maintaining their HIV treatment due to feelings of hopelessness or fear, ultimately harming their physical health and well-being.

## Contributing Factors to Internalized HIV Stigma

- **Societal Attitudes:** Myths, such as the idea that HIV is a consequence of moral failings, create a fertile ground for stigma. For instance, the enduring misconception that HIV only affects certain groups can isolate individuals and reinforce stigma.

- **Media Representation:** Movies or TV shows that depict those with HIV as 'villains' or as tragically doomed can influence public perception and, consequently, how individuals see themselves.

- **Cultural and Religious Beliefs:** In some cultures or religious communities, having HIV may be seen as a 'punishment,' which can deepen the internalized stigma, making people feel judged by their community.

- **Lack of Education:** Misunderstandings about HIV, such as the belief that it can be transmitted by casual contact, can drive fear and stigma. Even within healthcare settings, if professionals are not up-to-date on current HIV knowledge, they may unintentionally contribute to the stigma.

## Moving Forward: Combatting Internalized HIV Stigma

- **Educational Campaigns:** Providing accurate information about HIV to the public can dispel myths. For example, explaining that with proper treatment, HIV is a manageable chronic condition.

- **Positive Media Engagement:** Encouraging and supporting media to portray those with HIV in a realistic and positive light can help shift public perception.

- **Cultural Sensitivity Training:** Offering training for healthcare providers on cultural competence can help them support patients without reinforcing stigma.

- **Supportive Networks:** Establishing support groups where individuals with HIV can share experiences and feel less isolated can bolster self-esteem and community.

By addressing these factors and fostering an environment of support and education, we can significantly reduce the burden of internalized HIV stigma and empower those affected to lead full, healthy lives.

**Recognizing the Signs of Internalized HIV Stigma:**

- **Avoidance of Medical Care:** For example, a person might miss multiple HIV treatment appointments or stop taking their antiretroviral medication regularly, potentially due to feelings of shame or fear.

- **Social Withdrawal:** This could manifest as declining invitations to social events, distancing oneself from friends or family, or not engaging in previously enjoyed activities.

- **Negative Self-Talk:** Individuals may express feelings of worthlessness or internalize societal stigma, saying things like, "I'm no longer the same person" or "I don't deserve happiness."

- **Depression and Anxiety:** Signs include persistent sadness, loss of interest in daily activities, or constant worrying, all of which are heightened by the stigma surrounding HIV.

**Strategies to Address Internalized HIV Stigma:**

- **Education and Awareness:** Educate about HIV to debunk myths. For instance, explaining how modern treatments allow individuals to live long, healthy lives.

- **Empowerment Through Information:** Provide resources that highlight the successes and normalcy of living with HIV. For example, stories of people thriving with HIV can be inspiring.

- **Support Groups:** Facilitate groups where individuals share experiences and coping strategies, like a community center hosting regular meetings for those living with HIV.

- **Counseling and Mental Health Support:** Access to therapists or counselors who specialize in chronic illness can help individuals process and combat internalized stigma.

- **Advocacy and Community Engagement:** Participate in campaigns or events that promote understanding and acceptance of HIV, helping to reduce community-wide stigma.

**Role of Healthcare Professionals:**

- **Empathetic Communication:** Approach conversations with understanding and without judgment, such as saying, "It's completely normal to feel overwhelmed, but we're here to support you."

- **Continuous Education:** Regularly update knowledge on HIV to provide current and comprehensive care, ensuring patients receive the latest information and treatment options.

- **Challenge Stigma:** Actively address and correct any HIV-related stigma in healthcare settings, setting a precedent of respect and understanding.

**Conclusion:** Internalized HIV stigma significantly impacts the mental and physical well-being of those living with the virus. By recognizing the signs and implementing proactive strategies like education, support, and advocacy, we can foster a more inclusive and supportive environment. Healthcare professionals play a key role in this effort, leading by example through empathetic care and continuous learning. By working together, it's possible to reduce the burden of stigma and improve the quality of life for individuals with HIV.

## Knowledge Check

Welcome to the Knowledge Check sections! These segments are designed to enhance your understanding and retention of key concepts discussed in our training. Each section presents a series of thought-provoking questions or problems that will challenge your grasp of the material. By engaging with these questions, you'll have the opportunity to reflect on what you've learned, apply your knowledge in practical scenarios, and deepen your comprehension of the subject matter. These checks are a vital part of the learning process, enabling you to consolidate your learning and identify areas where you may need further clarification or study. Let's dive in and explore these concepts further!

1. **Question:** How does internalized stigma affect an individual's willingness to seek and adhere to HIV treatment, and what can be done to counteract this?

**Answer:** Internalized stigma can lead to a decreased willingness to seek and adhere to HIV treatment due to feelings of shame, fear of disclosure, or a belief that they are undeserving of care. For example, an individual might skip medication doses or avoid medical appointments to not confront their HIV status. To counteract this, healthcare providers can create a supportive environment that emphasizes confidentiality, provides empathetic counseling, and educates about the effectiveness of HIV treatments. Encouraging participation in support groups where individuals can share experiences and strategies for adherence can also be beneficial.

2. **Question:** What role does negative self-talk play in internalized HIV stigma, and how can individuals be supported to overcome this?

**Answer:** Negative self-talk in internalized HIV stigma often manifests as individuals blaming themselves, feeling unworthy, or perceiving themselves as less valuable. This can lead to depression and isolation, exacerbating the stigma. To support individuals, mental health professionals can employ techniques like cognitive-behavioral therapy to challenge and reframe negative thoughts. For example, replacing thoughts like "I am a burden" with "I have a support system that cares about me" can be empowering.

Additionally, peer support groups can provide a platform for individuals to share experiences and learn positive self-talk strategies from others facing similar challenges.

3. **Question:** In what ways can healthcare professionals actively challenge HIV-related stigma within healthcare settings?

**Answer:** Healthcare professionals can challenge HIV-related stigma by educating themselves and others about HIV, using people-first language, and correcting misinformation. For instance, if a healthcare worker hears a colleague making a stigmatizing comment, they should address it by providing factual information about HIV and its transmission. They can also foster a stigma-free environment by treating individuals with HIV with the same respect and dignity as any other patient. This includes having open, non-judgmental conversations about their health and treatment, and reassuring them of confidentiality and support.

4. **Question:** How can community engagement and advocacy work to reduce internalized HIV stigma?

**Answer:** Community engagement and advocacy can play a significant role in reducing internalized HIV stigma by raising public awareness, changing societal attitudes, and empowering individuals with HIV. Activities like community workshops, public health campaigns, and storytelling initiatives that share the experiences of those living successfully with HIV can challenge widespread misconceptions. For example, an advocacy campaign that highlights individuals with HIV leading fulfilling lives can help to dismantle stereotypes and normalize the condition, thereby reducing the internalization of stigma.

These questions and answers are designed to test and enhance your understanding of internalized HIV stigma. They focus on practical applications and strategies that can be employed to address and mitigate the effects of this form of stigma, using real-life examples for better comprehension.

## Understanding and Addressing External HIV Stigma

This section serves as a guide for training aimed at comprehending and addressing the stigma associated with HIV. Our objective is to provide comprehensive knowledge about the origins and consequences of stigma surrounding HIV, and to present well-founded strategies for its mitigation and management. By engaging with this material, participants will gain the tools to not only recognize the manifestations of HIV-related stigma but also to actively participate in efforts to diminish its presence and foster a more supportive and inclusive environment.

**Understanding External HIV Stigma:**

**Definition:**

- External HIV stigma encompasses the negative attitudes, beliefs, and behaviors that others direct towards individuals living with HIV. This stigma is often rooted in misinformation, fear of contagion, and societal prejudices.

- *Example:* A person living with HIV might experience avoidance by friends or family due to misconceptions about how HIV is transmitted.

**Forms of Stigma:**

- External stigma manifests in various forms, such as social exclusion, discrimination in healthcare settings, workplace discrimination, and negative portrayal in media.

- *Examples:*

  - Social Exclusion: People living with HIV being intentionally left out of social gatherings.

  - Healthcare Discrimination: A healthcare provider hesitating to provide care or making judgmental comments.

  - Workplace Discrimination: An employer denying a job or promotion due to the individual's HIV status.

  - Media Portrayal: TV shows or news reports depicting those with HIV in a stereotypical or negative light.

## The Impact of External HIV Stigma:

### On Individuals:

- Stigma can lead to psychological distress, such as anxiety or depression, and social isolation, as individuals may withdraw from social interactions to avoid discrimination.

- It can also create reluctance to seek testing, treatment, and care, critically impacting health outcomes.

- Moreover, it affects self-esteem and mental health, leading to feelings of shame or worthlessness.

- *Example:* An individual might avoid attending social events or delay seeking medical help due to fear of being stigmatized.

### On Public Health:

- At a broader level, stigma hampers HIV prevention efforts. It creates barriers to accessing HIV-related services, including testing and treatment.

- This, in turn, can increase the risk of HIV transmission, as individuals who are unaware of their status or unable to access treatment are more likely to inadvertently spread the virus.

- *Example:* Community members might avoid getting tested for HIV due to fear of being judged or discriminated against if diagnosed, thereby potentially increasing the spread of HIV.

This training material aims to provide not only a theoretical understanding of external HIV stigma but also practical strategies to combat it, fostering an environment of support and inclusivity for individuals living with HIV.

**Historical and Cultural Context of HIV Stigma:**

**Evolution of Stigma**

We will now briefly examine the historical development and societal impacts of HIV/AIDS stigma, particularly from the 1980s to the present. It explores how early misconceptions and fears surrounding HIV/AIDS contributed to the stigma, especially in the context of the LGBTQ+ community, and examines the role of cultural influences, including religious beliefs and societal norms.

### Early Fears and Misconceptions:

- **Context:** In the 1980s, with the emergence of HIV/AIDS, it was mistakenly labeled as a "gay plague." This label stemmed from a lack of understanding and contributed to deep-seated misconceptions and fears.

- **Example:** Picture the early years of HIV/AIDS, a time of uncertainty and fear. Due to limited knowledge, people hastily and incorrectly associated HIV with the gay community. This led to widespread stigma, with people hastily forming judgments based on fear rather than facts.

- **Impact on Individuals:** Every person diagnosed with HIV, irrespective of their sexual orientation, encountered societal rejection and fear.

- **Personal Example:** Consider someone like John, who, upon being diagnosed with HIV in the 1980s, faced not just the challenge of a serious health condition but also the heavy burden of social isolation and stigma.

**Cultural Influences**

### Role of Religious Beliefs:

- **Context:** In various cultures, religious beliefs significantly influenced attitudes towards HIV, at times framing it as a consequence of moral 'failings.'

- **Example:** Maria, from a religious community, faced immense internal conflict and fear of judgment when seeking help for her HIV condition, as her community viewed it as a result of moral lapse.

### Societal Norms and Stigma:

- **Context:** Societal norms that stigmatize behaviors like drug use or non-heteronormative sexual relationships have perpetuated HIV stigma.

- **Example:** Alex, who acquired HIV through intravenous drug use, struggled to find supportive services due to the stigma surrounding drug addiction. His experience highlights how societal attitudes can create barriers to seeking and receiving care.

Understanding the historical and cultural context of HIV stigma is vital. The initial fears and misconceptions of the 1980s have had a lasting impact, and cultural influences continue to affect perceptions and attitudes toward HIV/AIDS. By acknowledging and learning from these historical contexts, we can foster more empathetic and informed responses, reduce stigma, and provide more inclusive and understanding support to those affected by HIV/AIDS.

**Identifying External HIV Stigma:**

- **Recognizing Stigma in Settings:** Offer guidelines to identify stigma in healthcare (like reluctance to treat HIV patients), workplace (such as jokes about HIV), family (avoiding discussions about HIV), and community (excluding HIV-positive individuals from social events).

- **Subtle Stigma Forms:** Encourage awareness of less obvious stigma, like over-sympathizing with HIV-positive individuals or avoiding personal topics with them, which can feel patronizing or exclusionary.

**Strategies for Reducing External HIV Stigma:**

- **Education and Awareness:** Use real-life examples, such as correcting myths that HIV can be transmitted through casual contact, to promote understanding and reduce fear.

- **Advocacy and Policy Change:** Highlight successful policy changes, like the removal of HIV travel bans, and advocate for workplace anti-discrimination policies.

- **Community Engagement:** Encourage community forums or local HIV awareness events that foster dialogue and understanding.

- **Empowering People Living with HIV:** Share stories of individuals with HIV who have become advocates or public speakers challenging stigma.

**Role of Healthcare Professionals:**

- **Creating a Stigma-Free Environment:** Suggest practical steps like using inclusive language, displaying informative posters in clinics, and integrating HIV education into routine care.

**Practical Exercises:**

- **Interactive Learning:** Incorporate role-plays where participants handle scenarios of stigma in a healthcare setting or facilitate group discussions on personal experiences and perceptions of HIV stigma.

**Resources and Support:**

- **Further Learning and Support:** Provide a list of organizations, like the World Health Organization or local HIV support groups, and resources such as educational websites and community forums.

**Conclusion:**

This training document serves as a vital resource for those aiming to comprehend and effectively address HIV-related stigma. By adopting and implementing the strategies outlined herein, individuals, healthcare professionals, and community members can make a substantial impact. Their efforts will not only elevate the quality of life for those living with HIV but also contribute to broader public health advancements. Embracing these practices fosters a more inclusive and understanding environment, crucial for overcoming the challenges associated with HIV stigma and paving the way for better health outcomes and community well-being.

## Knowledge Check

Welcome to the Knowledge Check sections! These segments are designed to enhance your understanding and retention of key concepts discussed in our training. Each section presents a series of thought-provoking questions or problems that will challenge your grasp of the material. By engaging with these questions, you'll have the opportunity to reflect on what you've learned, apply your knowledge in practical scenarios, and deepen your comprehension of the subject matter. These checks are a vital part of the learning process, enabling you to consolidate your learning and identify areas where you may need further clarification or study. Let's dive in and explore these concepts further!

1. **Question:** How does external stigma affect the mental health of individuals living with HIV? Provide an example of a situation where this might occur.

**Best Answer:** External stigma can significantly impact the mental health of individuals living with HIV by fostering feelings of shame, isolation, and anxiety. For example, if a person living with HIV overhears colleagues making derogatory comments about HIV, they may feel isolated and fearful of disclosing their status, leading to increased stress and potentially depression. This situation exemplifies how societal attitudes and misconceptions can exacerbate the emotional burden on individuals with HIV, contributing to a decline in mental well-being.

2. **Question:** In what ways can external stigma create barriers to accessing healthcare for individuals living with HIV?

**Best Answer:** External stigma can create barriers to healthcare access through discrimination and judgment from healthcare providers and the community. For instance, if a person living with HIV perceives or experiences stigma from medical staff, they might avoid seeking timely medical care or be reluctant to disclose their status, leading to suboptimal treatment. This illustrates how stigma can directly impact the health outcomes of individuals with HIV by limiting their access to necessary medical care and support.

3. **Question:** How can external HIV stigma be challenged and reduced in a workplace setting?

**Best Answer:** Challenging and reducing external HIV stigma in the workplace involves creating an inclusive and informed environment. This can be achieved by implementing comprehensive education programs that dispel myths about HIV transmission and emphasize the importance of empathy and confidentiality. Additionally, enforcing anti-discrimination policies and providing support for employees living with HIV are crucial steps. An example would be a company hosting workshops on HIV awareness, highlighting the importance of inclusivity and support for all employees, regardless of their HIV status.

4. **Question:** What role do media and popular culture play in perpetuating external HIV stigma, and how can they be part of the solution?

**Best Answer:** Media and popular culture often perpetuate external HIV stigma through inaccurate representations and sensationalism, reinforcing misconceptions and fear. For example, a TV show that portrays a character with HIV as dangerous or unclean can reinforce harmful stereotypes. To be part of the solution, media and popular culture need to present informed, sensitive portrayals of individuals living with HIV, focusing on their diverse experiences and challenging existing stigmas. This approach can educate the public, normalize HIV, and contribute to a more accepting society.

5. **Question:** Discuss the impact of external HIV stigma on the willingness of individuals to get tested for HIV.

**Best Answer:** External HIV stigma can significantly deter individuals from getting tested for HIV, primarily due to fear of judgment or social repercussions if diagnosed positive. For instance, in a community where there is a high level of stigma associated with HIV, individuals might fear the social implications of a positive result, leading to avoidance of testing and late diagnosis. This demonstrates how stigma can act as a barrier to early detection and treatment, which is crucial for effective management of HIV and reducing its transmission.

## Understanding and Addressing HIV Stigma by Association

This resource is meticulously crafted to offer an in-depth understanding of the stigma by association with HIV. It delves into recognizing the subtle and overt signs of this stigma, delineating its features, and outlining effective methods to counteract it. Tailored for healthcare professionals, community advocates, and all those committed to eradicating the stigmatization associated with HIV, this guide serves as a valuable tool for fostering a more inclusive and supportive environment for individuals impacted by HIV.

**What is HIV-Related Stigma by Association?**

**Definition:**

Stigma by association with HIV refers to the negative beliefs and behaviors directed at individuals who are connected to people living with HIV (PLHIV), irrespective of their own HIV status. This stigma can impact friends, family members, healthcare workers, and community members.

**Examples for Clarity:**

- A family member of a person living with HIV might be unfairly excluded from social gatherings due to others' fears of HIV transmission.

- Healthcare providers might experience colleagues treating them differently because they work closely with PLHIV.

- Members of a community may face discrimination simply because they live in an area with a higher prevalence of HIV.

**Origins and Context:**

- Such stigma often arises from misunderstandings about how HIV is transmitted, leading to unnecessary fear and avoidance behaviors.

- Social fears and myths, such as the incorrect belief that HIV can spread through casual contact, fuel this type of stigma.

- Stereotypes in media representations and historical prejudices against groups disproportionately affected by HIV/AIDS contribute to stigma by association.

**Addressing Stigma by Association:**

- Education is key. Providing accurate information about HIV transmission can dispel myths and reduce fear.

- Advocacy and raising awareness about HIV can challenge societal stereotypes and change negative attitudes.

- Creating supportive networks for those affected by HIV, including their associates, fosters understanding and acceptance.

By employing person-first language and focusing on individuals' experiences, we can all contribute to a more supportive society for people impacted by HIV and their associates. This guide aims to be a step toward that compassionate and stigma-free future.

**Recognizing HIV Stigma by Association**

HIV stigma by association refers to negative attitudes and beliefs directed towards individuals who are closely connected to people living with HIV (PLHIV). Recognizing these stigmatizing behaviors is crucial for creating a more supportive and inclusive environment for everyone. Here are some key indicators, along with relatable examples, using person-first language:

**Social Isolation:**

- **Indicator:** Avoidance or distancing by friends or family from someone because of their connection to PLHIV.

- **Example:** John, whose brother is living with HIV, notices that his friends have stopped inviting him to gatherings. They may wrongly fear contracting HIV or feel uncomfortable due to misconceptions about the virus.

**Discriminatory Behaviors:**

- **Indicator:** Unfair treatment in workplaces, schools, or healthcare settings due to association with PLHIV.

- **Example:** Sarah, who volunteers at an HIV/AIDS support center, faces subtle discrimination at work. Her colleagues might exclude her from team lunches, mistakenly believing they can get HIV from casual contact.

**Stereotyping:**

- **Indicator:** Assuming someone has HIV because of their relationship with PLHIV.

- **Example:** Alex, who is dating someone living with HIV, experiences his peers jumping to conclusions that he must also be HIV-positive, despite HIV not being transmitted through casual contact or relationships.

**Language:**

- **Indicator:** Use of derogatory terms or insensitive phrases towards those associated with PLHIV.

- **Example:** Emma, a nurse who works in an HIV clinic, overhears people using stigmatizing language like "clean" or "dirty" to refer to individuals' HIV status or those associated with PLHIV.

## Situational Awareness:

- **Strategy:** Pay close attention to social dynamics and interactions in various environments.

- **Application:** In both personal and professional settings, be mindful of how people are treated based on their association with PLHIV. This could mean noticing if someone is consistently left out of social events or if there are changes in behavior towards them.

- **Strategy:** Be aware of subtle forms of discrimination and biases in everyday conversations.

- **Application:** Listen for and address misconceptions or insensitive jokes about HIV. Engaging in constructive conversations can help challenge and change these stigmatizing attitudes.

Understanding and recognizing HIV stigma by association is key to supporting and respecting not only people living with HIV but also those who are connected to them. This awareness helps foster a more inclusive and empathetic community.

## Characteristics of HIV Stigma by Association

Stigma associated with HIV continues to be a significant challenge, not only for people living with HIV (PLHIV) but also for those connected to them. This phenomenon, known as 'HIV stigma by association,' impacts friends, family members, caregivers, and even healthcare professionals who support PLHIV. Understanding the characteristics of this stigma is crucial in addressing its pervasive effects on individuals and communities. It involves recognizing and unpacking various forms of prejudice and misinformation that extend beyond the individuals directly affected by HIV. This introduction aims to shed light on these characteristics, providing insight into how they manifest and affect the daily lives and relationships of those indirectly experiencing the stigma surrounding HIV. By acknowledging and understanding these aspects, we can take significant steps towards fostering a more inclusive and empathetic society, where the burden of stigma is lifted, and supportive networks can thrive.

### Fear of Contagion:

- This involves the incorrect belief that HIV can be transmitted through everyday interactions, leading to an unfounded fear and avoidance of people associated with those living with HIV (PLHIV).

- **Example:** Imagine a scenario where someone hesitates to share a meal with a friend who has a family member living with HIV, wrongly believing they can catch the virus through shared utensils.

### Moral Judgment:

- This stigma stems from linking HIV with certain behaviors or lifestyles and then unfairly extending this judgment to those close to PLHIV.

- **Example:** A classic case would be a person being judged or looked down upon by neighbors simply because they regularly visit a sibling who is living with HIV, assuming incorrect lifestyle choices on both parts.

### Ignorance and Misinformation:

- This is about the lack of correct knowledge regarding how HIV is transmitted and treated, which leads to widespread misconceptions.

- **Example:** A co-worker might spread rumors and create fear in the workplace about a colleague who volunteers at an HIV clinic, due to their own misunderstandings about how HIV is transmitted.

### Invisibility:

- This aspect of stigma often remains unnoticed or unspoken, yet it acts as a silent and persistent barrier in the lives of those affected.

- **Example:** Consider a situation where family members of a person living with HIV receive fewer social invitations or community engagement opportunities, but this change is subtle and not openly discussed or acknowledged.

By understanding these characteristics with real-life examples, it becomes easier to recognize and address HIV stigma by association, helping to foster a more informed and compassionate community.


### Combating HIV Stigma by Association: A Person-First Approach

### Education and Awareness:

- Implement campaigns to educate about HIV, focusing on how it is and isn't transmitted. For example, a campaign could use simple animations to explain that HIV cannot be transmitted through casual contact like hugging or sharing utensils.

- Foster empathy and understanding towards people living with HIV (PLHIV) and their close contacts by sharing personal stories and experiences, illustrating the everyday lives and challenges faced by PLHIV.

### Encouraging Open Communication:

- Create forums or discussion groups, both online and in-person, where people can talk openly about HIV and stigma. These could be in the form of community meetings or virtual webinars.

- Urge individuals to share their own experiences or stories they've heard, creating a space that values honesty and vulnerability, thereby reducing stigma.

**Policy and Advocacy:**

- Advocate for laws and policies that safeguard the rights of PLHIV and their associates, ensuring they are free from discrimination. For instance, campaign for anti-discrimination policies in employment or housing for PLHIV.

- Strive to establish inclusive and equitable practices in workplaces, healthcare facilities, and communities, such as training sessions for staff on HIV and stigma.

**Support Networks:**

- Set up support groups specifically for friends and family members of PLHIV, offering a space to share experiences and receive advice. These could include regular meetings or an online forum for continuous support.

- Offer psychological and social support services, like counseling or social work assistance, to help those affected by stigma in managing their emotional and social well-being.

**Role Modeling and Leadership:**

- Encourage local leaders, celebrities, or influencers to publicly support PLHIV and denounce stigma. For example, a well-known local figure could share messages on social media or participate in public events supporting PLHIV.

- Lead by example, demonstrating respect and dignity in all interactions, regardless of someone's HIV status. This could be as simple as healthcare professionals showing equal care and attention to all patients, regardless of their HIV status.

Incorporating these strategies can significantly contribute to reducing HIV stigma by association, fostering a more understanding, inclusive, and empathetic society.

## Conclusion

Recognizing and effectively addressing the stigma associated with HIV is essential in fostering environments that are supportive, inclusive, and free from stigma. Education plays a pivotal role in dispelling the misconceptions and biases that perpetuate this form of stigma. By coupling advocacy with active community engagement, we have the power to dismantle these harmful stereotypes. This collective effort is the key to cultivating a society that is not only more understanding but also deeply empathetic towards individuals affected by HIV. The journey towards a stigma-free society begins with each of us taking proactive steps to challenge and change the narrative around HIV and its associated stigma.

Knowledge Check

Welcome to the Knowledge Check sections! These segments are designed to enhance your understanding and retention of key concepts discussed in our training. Each section presents a series of thought-provoking questions or problems that will challenge your grasp of the material. By engaging with these questions, you'll have the opportunity to reflect on what you've learned, apply your knowledge in practical scenarios, and deepen your comprehension of the subject matter. These checks are a vital part of the learning process, enabling you to consolidate your learning and identify areas where you may need further clarification or study. Let's dive in and explore these concepts further!

1. **Question:** How can stigma by association affect the family members of a person living with HIV?

**Answer:** Family members of a person living with HIV can experience stigma by association, which occurs when the stigma attached to HIV is transferred to them. This may manifest as social isolation, where friends or community members avoid them due to misconceptions about HIV transmission. For example, a family might be excluded from social gatherings, or their children might be treated differently at school. The key to addressing this is through education, emphasizing that HIV is not transmitted through casual contact and highlighting the importance of empathy and support for affected families.

2. **Question:** What role does the media play in perpetuating or combating HIV stigma by association?

**Answer:** The media has a significant impact on public perception and can either perpetuate or combat HIV stigma by association. When the media inaccurately portrays HIV as a condition only affecting certain groups or as highly contagious through casual contact, it fuels misconceptions and fear. However, when media outlets focus on factual, sensitive reporting and include stories of individuals living healthily and positively with HIV, it helps combat stigma. An example is a news feature that showcases the everyday life of a person with HIV, emphasizing their normal interactions and challenges unrelated to their HIV status, thereby normalizing their experience and reducing stigma by association.

3. **Question:** How can healthcare professionals inadvertently contribute to stigma by association in HIV, and what practices can they adopt to avoid this?

**Answer:** Healthcare professionals may unintentionally contribute to stigma by association through their language, attitudes, or policies that isolate and discriminate against people living with HIV. For example, a nurse expressing reluctance to treat a person with HIV or using excessive protective gear beyond standard precautions can reinforce fear and stigma. To avoid this, healthcare professionals should practice universal precautions uniformly with all patients, use people-first language, and offer the same level of care and empathy as they would to any other patient. Training in cultural competence and sensitivity towards HIV can also be instrumental in changing these behaviors.

4. **Question:** What are the potential psychological impacts on an individual who experiences HIV stigma by association, and what support can be offered?

**Answer:** Individuals experiencing HIV stigma by association may face psychological impacts such as anxiety, depression, and a feeling of isolation. They might feel unfairly judged due to their association with HIV, leading to stress and a diminished sense of self-worth. Support can be offered through counseling services, support groups where they can share experiences with others facing similar challenges, and community education programs that aim to reduce stigma. For instance, a support group can provide a safe space for family members of people with HIV to discuss their experiences and coping strategies.

These questions and answers provide a comprehensive understanding of HIV stigma by association, emphasizing the need for education, empathy, and supportive practices to combat this issue.

## Who Can you Tell?

### Introduction: Challenging the Shadows of Stigma

In the vibrant heart of New Orleans, where jazz notes weave through the air and the spirit of resilience dances in the streets, four fictitious lives intersected on a common journey - one that would forever change the way they saw HIV stigma. Each person brought a unique perspective, shedding light on the insidious ways stigma permeates society. As we journey through their stories, we invite you to reflect not only on the impact of stigma but also on your own power to combat it. These tales are a testament to the strength of the human spirit and a call to action, reminding us all that we have a choice to make. The question they leave us with is simple yet profound: Who Can You Tell? This paper was originally created to be presented at the International Conference on Stigma.

### Internalized Stigma - The Battle Within

Amelia sat on the balcony of her quaint New Orleans apartment, a jazz tune humming softly from the streets below. The warm breeze played with her hair as she gazed at the vibrant city that she had called home for so long. But behind her bright eyes hid a heavy secret - one that weighed down her soul more than the sultry Louisiana air ever could.

Amelia had been living with HIV for over a decade, and her battle was not just against the virus but against the relentless stigma that had crept into her own mind. Every morning, she faced the mirror, her own reflection becoming a silent judge. She scrutinized herself, dissecting every aspect of her life.

"I should have been more careful," she whispered to her reflection. "I should have protected myself. I should have avoided this."

It was the internalized stigma, the self-blame, that was the hardest to overcome. Amelia was a fierce advocate for HIV awareness in her community, but her toughest fight was with herself. The whispers of doubt haunted her even in her most intimate moments. The fear of rejection had become a constant companion.

As she looked out over the colorful houses and winding streets of the French Quarter, she couldn't help but yearn for the freedom to be herself without judgment. She longed for the day when she could look in the mirror and see not just her own reflection but the strength and resilience that had carried her through this journey.

## External Stigma - Judgement From the Outside

Continuing down the bustling streets of New Orleans, we come across Malik, a charismatic and talented street musician. With his guitar in hand and a voice that could melt even the coldest of hearts, he had always been a local favorite. Yet, despite his outward confidence, there was an unspoken pain that lingered beneath his smile.

Malik had recently disclosed his HIV status to a close friend, thinking that the burden of secrecy would finally be lifted. However, as word spread through the close-knit community like wildfire, he experienced external stigma like never before. Friends turned their backs, and strangers in the crowd would whisper when he walked by.

"Stay away from him; he's sick."

The snide comments and the alienation cut deeper than any insult he'd ever received. Malik felt the weight of external stigma press down on him like an oppressive humidity, even in the midst of a New Orleans summer.

Despite the rejection and ostracization, Malik refused to give in to despair. Every strum of his guitar and every note of his songs became a defiant statement, a declaration that his worth was not defined by the judgments of others. He played his music with an unyielding spirit, hoping that his melodies would one day drown out the voices of prejudice.

As he sang his heart out on the streets of the French Quarter, he knew that true change would only come when society learned to see beyond the virus, beyond the stigma, and recognize the humanity that resided in every person, regardless of their health status. Malik believed that New Orleans, with its soulful heart and resilient spirit, had the potential to lead this change and turn the page on the chapter of external stigma.

## Stigma by Association - The Ties That Bind

As the sun dipped below the Mississippi, casting a warm glow across the riverfront, we found ourselves in the company of Lila, a vivacious and compassionate young woman who worked at a local non-profit organization. Lila's brother, Daniel, had been living with HIV for years, and she had seen firsthand the discrimination he faced.

Lila watched as her brother withdrew from family gatherings, his once infectious laughter silenced by the fear of judgment. She could see the pain in his eyes, a pain that she herself felt as she witnessed the injustice of stigma by association. Her friends would warn her to keep her distance from her brother, fearing that they might also contract the virus through casual contact.

But Lila refused to let stigma tear her family apart. She had become an advocate not only for her brother but for all those living with HIV. She believed in the power of education, in dispelling the myths surrounding HIV transmission, and in forging a community that supported rather than shunned.

Lila organized workshops and support groups, inviting experts and survivors to share their stories. She knew that knowledge was the most potent weapon against stigma. She challenged her friends and acquaintances, patiently explaining that HIV was not transmitted through hugs, laughter, or shared meals.

Her tireless efforts began to make a difference. Slowly but surely, the cloud of stigma that had hung over her family and others living with HIV began to lift. She had turned her pain into a force for change.

Lila knew that as long as even one person continued to be stigmatized, her work was far from done. She dreamt of a New Orleans where love and acceptance would conquer fear and prejudice, and where no one would be judged by association.

**A Call to Action - Changing Hearts and Minds**

Amelia, Malik, and Lila, each carrying their own unique experiences of HIV-related stigma, found themselves united by a shared desire for change. Their stories, while distinct, converged into a collective call to action - a call that resonated not only in New Orleans but across the world.

Amelia had resolved to overcome her internalized stigma, to embrace self-love, and to use her experience as a beacon of hope for others. She began sharing her story, not just as an advocate but as a human being. She showed that living with HIV was not a moral failing but a medical condition, and that anyone could be affected. Through her vulnerability, she challenged stereotypes and invited empathy.

Malik, despite the external stigma he faced, refused to let it silence his music. Instead, he transformed his pain into melodies that told stories of resilience. His soulful tunes became anthems of courage, inspiring others to stand up against discrimination. He used his voice not only to sing but also to speak out against ignorance, reminding people that empathy was the antidote to stigma.

Lila, driven by her love for her brother and her unwavering belief in education, had become a bridge between those living with HIV and those who feared it. She organized workshops, support groups, and awareness campaigns. She emphasized that stigma not only hurt individuals but hindered efforts to combat the virus effectively. Lila was on a mission to show that compassion and knowledge could break the chains of ignorance.

Together, they formed a powerful alliance, and their stories reverberated through the heart of New Orleans and beyond. They spoke of acceptance, understanding, and unity, challenging a society that had long been blinded by prejudice. Their message was clear - it was time to change hearts and minds.

Their call to action extended to all who heard their stories. It was a call for communities to come together, for families to embrace their loved ones, and for individuals to educate themselves about HIV. It was a plea for empathy, a rejection of judgment, and an affirmation of the inherent worth of every human being.

In New Orleans, where music, culture, and diversity flowed through the streets like the mighty Mississippi River, they found the perfect backdrop for their movement. They knew that by joining forces, they could transform their city into a beacon of acceptance, a place where stigma would wither, and compassion would flourish.

Their stories were no longer just personal journeys; they had become the driving force behind a movement for change. As the sun set over the crescent city, it cast a warm light on a future where HIV stigma would be nothing more than a distant memory, and love, acceptance, and understanding would prevail.

# Introduction to Working with Justice-Involved and Justice-Impacted Individuals

Engaging with justice-involved and justice-impacted individuals presents a unique set of challenges, yet it offers a deeply rewarding opportunity for healthcare professionals. This population, having interacted with the criminal justice system either directly or indirectly, faces a distinctive blend of needs and obstacles that require a specialized approach to care.

**Understanding the Unique Needs and Challenges**

Justice-involved individuals often grapple with a history of incarceration, legal struggles, and the ongoing consequences of having a criminal record. These experiences can lead to profound stigma and discrimination in various aspects of life, including difficulties in securing employment, housing, and accessing healthcare services. For example, a person with a past conviction might find it nearly impossible to rent an apartment or may be repeatedly turned down for job opportunities, intensifying feelings of exclusion and hopelessness.

Similarly, justice-impacted individuals – those who have family members or close friends entangled in the justice system – face their own set of challenges. They may experience emotional strain, financial burdens, and social stigma by association. A child with an incarcerated parent, for instance, may confront bullying at school and struggle with emotional and behavioral issues.

**Enhanced Understanding of Working with Justice-Involved and Justice-Impacted Individuals**

When healthcare professionals engage with individuals who have interacted with the criminal justice system, a deep understanding of their unique experiences and challenges is crucial. This understanding spans two key areas: Justice Involvement and Justice Impact.

**Justice Involvement: A Broad Spectrum**

- **Arrests:** The experience of being arrested can be traumatic and may lead to distrust in systems of authority. For example, an individual who has been arrested may feel anxious during interactions with healthcare providers due to perceived power imbalances.

- **Convictions:** A conviction can lead to long-lasting stigma and alter an individual's self-identity. Healthcare providers might encounter patients who feel defined by their conviction, impacting their self-esteem and mental health.

- **Incarceration:** Time spent in incarceration can significantly impact physical and mental health. Incarcerated individuals may experience issues such as inadequate healthcare, exposure to communicable diseases, or psychological distress from isolation.

### Justice Impact: The Ripple Effect

- **Employment Loss:** Post-incarceration, finding employment can be a major hurdle due to societal stigma. Healthcare professionals might encounter individuals dealing with the stress and anxiety of unemployment, affecting their overall health.

- **Housing Instability:** The challenge of securing stable housing post-release can lead to homelessness or unsafe living conditions, exacerbating health issues.

- **Family Relationships:** Incarceration can strain family dynamics, leading to emotional distress. A healthcare provider may need to address issues like depression or anxiety stemming from family separation or conflict.

- **Stigma:** The stigma associated with being justice-involved can lead to social isolation and marginalization, negatively impacting mental health. Healthcare providers should be sensitive to this and create a non-judgmental environment.

- **Mental Health Issues:** The trauma of criminal justice system involvement often leads to mental health challenges such as PTSD, depression, or anxiety. A patient's history of justice involvement should prompt healthcare providers to screen for these conditions.

- **Substance Abuse:** There is a high prevalence of substance use disorders among justice-involved individuals. Providers should be prepared to offer or refer patients to appropriate substance abuse treatment programs.

### Cultivating a Culturally Competent and Trauma-Informed Approach

To effectively work with this population, healthcare professionals must cultivate a culturally competent and trauma-informed approach. This involves understanding the socio-cultural backgrounds of these individuals and recognizing how their experiences with the justice system have shaped their perspectives and health needs.

A culturally competent approach means being sensitive to the diverse cultural, ethnic, and social backgrounds of justice-involved individuals. For example, understanding the specific challenges faced by individuals from minority communities who may experience systemic biases in the justice system can help in tailoring more effective and empathetic care strategies.

A trauma-informed approach is equally crucial. Many justice-involved individuals have experienced trauma, whether from encounters with law enforcement, the conditions of incarceration, or the challenges of reintegration into society. Recognizing signs of trauma, such as anxiety, depression, or substance abuse, and responding with appropriate care can make a significant difference. For instance, when a healthcare provider encounters a patient exhibiting signs of PTSD, acknowledging this as a potential consequence of their justice involvement can lead to more effective, tailored treatment plans.

### Navigating the Challenges of Stigma and Discrimination for Justice-Involved Individuals

Working with justice-involved individuals presents unique challenges, particularly in addressing the pervasive stigma and discrimination they often face. As healthcare professionals, it's vital to understand these challenges in depth and develop strategies to help individuals overcome them. Below are key areas where stigma and discrimination manifest, along with detailed examples and practical mitigation strategies.

**Stigma and Discrimination in Various Aspects of Life:**

### In Employment:

- **Challenge:** Individuals with criminal records frequently encounter barriers in the job market. For example, someone with a history of theft may find doors to retail jobs closed, significantly restricting their job prospects. Even when opportunities arise, they often involve low-wage or unstable positions, hindering long-term stability and growth.

- **Mitigation Strategies:** Healthcare professionals can guide these individuals towards job training and placement programs tailored for justice-involved persons. Additionally, they can collaborate with employment agencies that focus on high-demand skills training, thereby increasing employability in stable, well-paying sectors.

### In Housing:

- **Challenge:** Obtaining stable housing is a significant challenge, as landlords and housing authorities often perform background checks. A criminal record can lead to repeated rejections, pushing individuals towards homelessness or unstable living situations like temporary shelters.

- **Mitigation Strategies:** Professionals can refer individuals to housing assistance programs specifically designed for those with criminal records. They can also advocate for their clients with local housing authorities or non-profit organizations that provide supportive housing solutions.

### In Social Interactions:

- **Challenge:** Social exclusion and judgment are common, making it difficult for justice-involved individuals to build supportive social networks. For instance, community members might keep their distance from someone known to have a criminal history, hindering their social reintegration and access to informal support networks.

- **Mitigation Strategies:** Encourage participation in community activities that foster inclusivity, such as volunteer projects or local events. Facilitate connections with support groups where individuals can share experiences and receive peer support. Educating the broader community on the challenges faced by justice-involved individuals can also help reduce stigma.

### In Healthcare Settings:

- **Challenge:** Within healthcare settings, justice-involved individuals may face biases and judgment from staff, impacting their access to quality care.

- **Mitigation Strategies:** Training healthcare providers in cultural competency and trauma-informed care is crucial. Creating a non-judgmental, supportive environment in healthcare settings can significantly improve care outcomes for these individuals.

As healthcare professionals, understanding the depth of challenges faced by justice-involved individuals is the first step towards meaningful support. By acknowledging and actively working to mitigate the effects of stigma and discrimination in employment, housing, social interactions, and healthcare settings, professionals can play a pivotal role in aiding the reintegration and overall well-being of these individuals. Building partnerships with community organizations, advocating for policy changes, and educating the public and healthcare providers about these challenges can collectively contribute to more inclusive and supportive communities.

**Addressing Trauma in Justice-Involved Individuals**

Healthcare professionals play a crucial role in addressing the complex needs of justice-involved individuals. A significant aspect of their care involves understanding and mitigating the impact of trauma. For these individuals, trauma is not just a single event but often a series of life-altering experiences that can profoundly affect their mental and physical health. Here, we delve into the types of trauma they may face, the potential for substance abuse as a coping mechanism, and strategies for effective trauma-informed care.

**Understanding and Addressing Exposure to Violence in Justice-Involved Individuals**

Justice-involved individuals often have a history of direct or indirect exposure to violence. This exposure can manifest in various forms, such as physical altercations, witnessing violent acts, or being victims of abuse. Such experiences can have profound psychological effects, potentially leading to conditions like Post-Traumatic Stress Disorder (PTSD).

**Types of Violence Exposure and Their Impacts:**

**Physical Altercations:**

- **Example:** An individual who has been involved in or witnessed frequent fights or physical assaults may develop heightened aggression or fear responses.

- **Impact:** They might exhibit hypervigilance, a common symptom of PTSD, where they are constantly on edge, anticipating danger.

**Witnessing Violence:**

- **Example:** Observing acts of violence, such as community or domestic violence, can lead to feelings of helplessness and fear.

- **Impact:** Such individuals might develop anxiety disorders, experience nightmares, or have flashbacks of these events.

**Victims of Abuse:**

- **Example:** Experiencing abuse, whether physical, emotional, or sexual, particularly in formative years, can deeply impact mental health.

- **Impact:** This can lead to issues like depression, anxiety, trust issues, and in severe cases, dissociative disorders.

## Strategies for Healthcare Professionals:

### Trauma-Informed Care:

- Recognize signs of trauma in behavior and communication. For instance, a patient who avoids eye contact or seems excessively wary might be displaying trauma-related behavior.

- Create a safe and non-judgmental environment where patients feel comfortable sharing their experiences.

### Building Trust:

- Develop a rapport through consistent, respectful interactions. Show empathy and understanding towards their experiences.

- Use active listening skills to validate their feelings and experiences. For example, acknowledging the difficulty of discussing past abuse can foster trust.

### Individualized Care Plans:

- Develop care plans that address specific trauma-related issues. For instance, for someone with a history of domestic violence, include counseling services specializing in domestic abuse.

- Collaborate with other professionals, like psychologists or social workers, for a holistic approach to treatment.

### Educating and Empowering Patients:

- Educate patients about the effects of trauma on mental and physical health. Use relatable examples, like explaining how chronic stress from past violence can impact physical health.

- Empower them with coping strategies and resources. Teach relaxation techniques or refer them to support groups where they can connect with others with similar experiences.

### Cultural Sensitivity:

- Understand how cultural backgrounds can influence the perception of and reaction to violence. Some cultures might stigmatize the discussion of certain types of violence, like domestic abuse.

- Approach such topics with cultural sensitivity and respect for their background and beliefs.

### Regular Follow-Ups:

- Schedule regular follow-ups to monitor their progress and make any necessary adjustments to their care plan.

- Use these sessions to reassess their emotional and physical well-being, and to provide continuous support.

Working with justice-involved individuals who have experienced violence requires a compassionate, trauma-informed approach. By recognizing the specific types of violence exposure and its impacts, healthcare professionals can develop effective, individualized care strategies. Building trust, providing education, and ensuring cultural sensitivity are key in supporting these individuals towards recovery and improved well-being.

## Addressing and Understanding Emotional and Psychological Abuse

When working with individuals who have been justice-involved or justice-impacted, it's crucial to recognize that trauma can manifest in various forms, not just physical. Emotional and psychological abuse, often less visible, can have profound and lasting effects on an individual's mental health and well-being.

### Definition and Examples:

- Emotional and psychological abuse involves behaviors that harm an individual's sense of self-worth or emotional well-being. Examples include constant criticism, humiliation, gaslighting (making someone doubt their reality), and isolating an individual from friends and family.

- In a justice-involved context, this might include being constantly undermined by authorities, or for justice-impacted individuals, dealing with the social stigma of having a family member in the criminal justice system.

### Identifying the Signs:

- Symptoms of emotional abuse might include severe anxiety, depression, post-traumatic stress disorder (PTSD), or a pervasive sense of mistrust in others.

- For example, an individual who has been repeatedly belittled may exhibit extreme self-doubt in decision-making or feel unworthy of positive attention and support.

### Strategies for Healthcare Professionals:

### Building Trust:

- Establishing a trusting relationship is crucial. Start by creating a safe and non-judgmental space for individuals to share their experiences.

- Example: A healthcare provider might begin a session by reassuring the individual that their feelings and experiences are valid and that the space is confidential and supportive.

**Active Listening and Validation:**

- Engage in active listening, giving full attention to the individual, and validate their feelings and experiences.
- For instance, if a justice-impacted individual expresses feelings of isolation due to a family member's incarceration, acknowledge the difficulty of their situation and the strength it takes to cope with such challenges.

**Empowerment and Self-Esteem Building:**

- Encourage and support activities that build self-esteem. This could include goal-setting, affirmations, or engaging in new skills or hobbies.
- A practical example would be guiding an individual to engage in community activities or groups that align with their interests, fostering a sense of achievement and belonging.

**Cognitive Behavioral Therapy (CBT):**

- CBT can be particularly effective in addressing the negative thought patterns associated with emotional abuse.
- For example, through CBT, an individual who has experienced manipulation may learn to recognize and challenge distorted beliefs they have developed about themselves.

**Trauma-Informed Care:**

- Understand and acknowledge the impact of trauma on an individual's life and offer care that is sensitive to these experiences.
- This might involve being aware of triggers and working collaboratively with the individual to develop coping strategies.

**Referrals to Specialized Services:**

- In cases where specialized intervention is required, such as severe anxiety or PTSD, refer to mental health professionals who have expertise in treating trauma resulting from emotional and psychological abuse.
- Collaboration with social workers or counselors who have experience working with justice-involved and justice-impacted individuals can also be beneficial.

Working with individuals who have experienced emotional and psychological abuse, especially in the context of justice involvement, requires a compassionate, patient, and holistic approach. By recognizing the signs, employing effective communication strategies, and providing appropriate support and referrals, healthcare professionals can play a pivotal role in facilitating healing and empowerment for these individuals.

**Understanding Incarceration Experiences:**

Incarceration is not just a physical confinement; it's an experience that can fundamentally alter a person's psychological and emotional state. Healthcare professionals need to understand the multifaceted impact of incarceration to provide effective care for this population.

### Trauma of Incarceration:

- The abrupt loss of autonomy and freedom can be deeply traumatic. Individuals might experience feelings of powerlessness, fear, and anxiety.

- Exposure to potentially hostile or violent environments can lead to chronic stress or post-traumatic stress disorder (PTSD).

- The stress of adjusting to the rigid and often dehumanizing routines of prison life can exacerbate existing mental health issues or trigger new ones.

### Examples to Consider:

- A person who has experienced violence or threats within the prison may develop hypervigilance, a constant state of alertness that doesn't subside even after release.

- The isolation experienced, especially in solitary confinement, can lead to severe anxiety, depression, or worsen existing mental health conditions.

- The stigma of being incarcerated can continue to impact an individual's self-esteem and mental health long after their release.

## Strategies for Healthcare Professionals:

### Trauma-Informed Care:

- Recognize signs of trauma, such as withdrawal, aggression, or anxiety, and approach care with sensitivity to these experiences.

- Create a safe, non-judgmental space where individuals feel comfortable discussing their experiences.

### Building Trust:

- Understand that trust may be difficult to establish due to negative experiences with authority figures in the prison system.

- Be consistent, transparent, and patient in interactions to gradually build a trusting relationship.

### Comprehensive Assessment:

- Conduct thorough assessments to understand the full extent of the impact of incarceration, including physical health, mental health, and social well-being.

- Recognize that some health issues might be direct results of prison conditions, such as poor nutrition or exposure to infectious diseases.

### Cultural Competency:

- Acknowledge and respect the diverse backgrounds of justice-involved individuals, understanding that experiences and perceptions of incarceration can vary greatly across different cultures and communities.

### Support for Reintegration:

- Assist with access to services that support reintegration, such as job training, housing assistance, and reconnecting with family.

- Understand that reintegration is a gradual process and offer continued support and follow-up care.

### Collaborative Care Approach:

- Work collaboratively with other professionals, such as social workers, mental health therapists, and community organizations, to provide a holistic approach to care.

- Facilitate connections to community resources that can assist with various needs, from employment to mental health services.

Working with individuals who have experienced incarceration requires a deep understanding of the complex and often traumatic nature of their experiences. By employing trauma-informed, culturally competent, and patient-centered approaches, healthcare professionals can significantly aid in the healing and reintegration process of justice-involved individuals. It's crucial to recognize that the journey to recovery and reintegration is unique for each individual and requires a compassionate, multi-faceted approach to care.

## Substance Abuse as a Coping Mechanism

Working with justice-involved and justice-impacted individuals requires a deep understanding of the complex factors that influence their experiences with the criminal justice system. These individuals often navigate a multitude of challenges, including social stigma, reintegration into society, and dealing with the long-lasting effects of their experiences. Healthcare professionals in this field must develop a nuanced approach, characterized by empathy, cultural sensitivity, and an awareness of the specific needs and histories of these individuals. This section aims to delve into some of the key issues, such as substance abuse as a coping mechanism, and provide practical strategies and examples to aid healthcare professionals in effectively supporting this population.

### Understanding Self-Medication:

### Background and Context:

- Many justice-involved and justice-impacted individuals have encountered significant trauma, whether through direct experiences with the criminal justice system or through the repercussions of a loved one's involvement.

- To cope with the stress, anxiety, and emotional pain stemming from these experiences, some turn to substance use as a form of self-medication.

**The Cycle of Dependency:**

- Initially, substances may seem to offer a temporary reprieve from emotional and psychological distress. For example, a person with a history of incarceration might use alcohol to numb feelings of shame or isolation.

- However, this relief is fleeting and often leads to a dangerous cycle of dependency. As tolerance builds, the individual may consume more, increasing the risk of addiction.

**Compounding Challenges:**

- Substance abuse adds layers of complexity to an already challenging situation. For instance, an individual using substances to cope with the trauma of witnessing violence in prison might find themselves struggling with health issues, strained relationships, and difficulties in maintaining employment.

**Understanding and Addressing the Lack of Support**

Working with justice-involved and justice-impacted individuals presents a unique set of challenges and opportunities for healthcare professionals. This population often contends with a myriad of issues stemming from their involvement with the criminal justice system, which can significantly affect their health and well-being. As a healthcare provider, understanding these challenges and employing effective strategies to address them is not just beneficial – it's essential for fostering successful reintegration and improving health outcomes. Expect to touch on the following areas with your client.

**Financial Challenges:**

- **Scenario:** Upon release, an individual might have no immediate income source, making it difficult to afford essentials like food or transportation.

- **Healthcare Role:** Professionals can guide them to local food banks, low-cost transportation services, or emergency financial aid programs.

**Job Training and Education:**

- **Scenario:** An individual may have never completed high school or lacks vocational skills, limiting their employment opportunities.

- **Healthcare Role:** Refer them to adult education classes or vocational training programs. Healthcare facilities could collaborate with local community colleges or trade schools.

**Healthcare Access:**

- **Scenario:** Many lack health insurance or are unaware of free or sliding-scale clinics, hindering access to necessary medical, mental health, or substance abuse treatment.

- **Healthcare Role:** Provide information about Medicaid or local clinics offering low-cost services. Partner with mental health providers who specialize in trauma-informed care for this demographic.

**Mitigation Strategies:**

- **Collaborative Efforts:** Create partnerships with social workers and community organizations to establish a comprehensive support network.

- **Advocacy:** Advocate for policies that facilitate access to healthcare, such as extending Medicaid coverage or funding community health programs tailored to this group.

## Empowering Through Active Support and Understanding

For healthcare professionals, the journey starts with recognizing the unique barriers faced by justice-involved individuals. By creating an environment that is both supportive and non-judgmental, professionals can not only address immediate health concerns but also assist in the broader aspects of reintegration. For instance, by simply having a list of local resources at hand - from job centers to mental health support groups - healthcare providers can offer more than just medical care; they can offer hope and direction.

Involvement doesn't end with referrals. Following up on these recommendations, understanding the progress, and adjusting the support as needed are vital. For example, if an individual is struggling with a specific training program, the healthcare provider might explore alternative educational resources or support services that better align with their needs and capabilities.

In essence, the role of healthcare professionals in this context is multifaceted. It's not just about treating physical ailments but also about understanding the social determinants of health that affect this population. By employing empathy, providing targeted referrals, and advocating for systemic changes, healthcare professionals can significantly impact the lives of justice-involved and justice-impacted individuals, aiding in their journey towards a healthier and more stable life.

## Being an Advocate:

As a healthcare professional, your advocacy can make a significant difference in the lives of justice-involved and justice-impacted individuals. Advocacy involves not just medical care, but also standing up for the rights and needs of these individuals in broader societal contexts. Here's how:

- ❖ **Understanding Systemic Barriers:** Recognize that justice-involved individuals often face systemic barriers in areas like employment and housing due to their criminal records. For example, an individual with a minor drug offense might struggle to find housing because many landlords conduct background checks, leading to automatic disqualification.

- ❖ **Promoting Inclusive Policies:** Advocate for inclusive hiring practices within your organization. Encourage policies that provide equal opportunities to justice-involved individuals. For instance, support the implementation of 'Ban the Box' policies in job applications, which remove the checkbox asking if applicants have a criminal record. This allows candidates to be judged first on their qualifications.

❖ **Educational Sessions:** Organize educational sessions for employers and landlords to inform them about the challenges faced by justice-involved individuals and how supporting their reintegration benefits the community. Use relatable examples, like the success stories of individuals who rebuilt their lives post-incarceration, to highlight the positive outcomes of such support.

## Policy Change and Community Engagement:

✓ **Policy Advocacy:** Engage in policy advocacy by supporting legislation that aids the reintegration of justice-involved individuals. This could involve writing to local representatives, participating in advocacy groups, or speaking at public forums. Emphasize the public health benefits of successful reintegration, such as reduced recidivism and improved community health outcomes.

✓ **Community Partnerships:** Develop partnerships with local businesses and organizations to create employment opportunities for justice-involved individuals. For example, collaborate with a local cafe to set up a barista training program for individuals with a criminal record, offering both skill development and employment opportunities.

✓ **Healthcare Policy Reform:** Advocate for healthcare policy reform that addresses the specific needs of justice-involved individuals. This could include increased funding for mental health services, substance abuse treatment programs, or healthcare services within correctional facilities.

✓ **Educational Advocacy:** Work towards incorporating education about the justice system and its impact on health into medical school curricula and continuing education for healthcare professionals. This ensures that upcoming and current healthcare professionals are better equipped to understand and address the unique healthcare needs of this population.

Advocacy for justice-involved and justice-impacted individuals is a multifaceted responsibility that extends beyond the healthcare setting. It involves understanding systemic barriers, actively working towards policy change, and fostering community partnerships. By taking these steps, healthcare professionals can play a crucial role in supporting the reintegration of these individuals into society, thereby contributing to healthier and more inclusive communities.

## Conclusion

Healthcare professionals play a pivotal role in supporting the reintegration and well-being of justice-involved and justice-impacted individuals. By approaching care with empathy, respect, cultural awareness, and an understanding of trauma, they can significantly improve health outcomes and facilitate a smoother transition into society for these individuals. Remember, the goal is not just to treat immediate health concerns but also to empower them towards a healthier, more stable future.

# Introduction to Trauma-Informed Care

Trauma-Informed Care (TIC) represents a comprehensive approach to service delivery, deeply acknowledging and responding to the extensive impact of trauma on an individual's life. This method emphasizes the recognition and understanding of trauma symptoms and their potential role in shaping a person's experiences and responses. The importance of TIC is underscored by the fact that a substantial majority, over 90%, of individuals in behavioral healthcare settings have reported experiencing trauma. The implications of trauma are far-reaching, profoundly influencing not just mental health but also physical, emotional, social, and spiritual aspects of well-being. By adopting TIC, service providers can more effectively support individuals on their journey of recovery, offering care that is not only sensitive to but also shaped by an understanding of these traumatic experiences. This approach is crucial in fostering healing and resilience, ensuring that care systems are not merely responsive but also proactive in addressing the multifaceted needs of those affected by trauma.

**Understanding Trauma and Its Effects**

Trauma transcends the mere occurrence of distressing events; it encompasses the unique emotional and psychological reactions individuals have to these experiences. The subjective nature of trauma is such that two people might undergo an identical event, like a car accident or a catastrophic natural event, yet their emotional responses and enduring effects can vary significantly. This variation underscores the personal aspect of trauma, shaped by individual perceptions, past experiences, and coping mechanisms.

Sources of trauma are manifold, encompassing experiences like childhood abuse, domestic violence, sexual assault, military combat, and exposure to natural disasters, among others. The diversity of these sources highlights that trauma can arise from both one-time events and ongoing, chronic situations.

The ramifications of trauma are extensive and multifaceted, affecting individuals on multiple levels. Psychological responses can include persistent feelings of anxiety and depression, often reflecting the internal turmoil and struggle to process the traumatic event. Additionally, some individuals might turn to substance abuse as a coping mechanism, attempting to self-medicate the distressing emotions and memories associated with their trauma.

A particularly profound impact of trauma is the development of post-traumatic stress disorder (PTSD), a condition characterized by intense, disturbing thoughts and feelings related to their traumatic experiences that persist long after the event has ended. Individuals with PTSD may relive the trauma through flashbacks or nightmares; they may feel sadness, fear, anger, and detached or estranged from other people.

Understanding trauma's deep and varied impacts is crucial for recognizing the need for a personalized approach to treatment and support. It necessitates acknowledging that each individual's journey through trauma and recovery is unique, shaped by a complex interplay of personal history, resilience, and current life circumstances.

**Principles of Trauma-Informed Care:**

Understanding the principles of trauma-informed care is essential for creating a therapeutic environment that promotes healing and empowerment. Here are the principles, each elaborated with detailed examples to deepen understanding and provide context:

- **Safety:** The cornerstone of trauma-informed care is the assurance of both physical and emotional safety. For example, in a therapy setting, this might mean arranging the seating to ensure that clients are not startled by someone entering the room. It could also involve establishing clear boundaries at the outset, such as the client knowing they can take a break from a session if they feel overwhelmed. In a broader context, emotional safety might mean that a support group leader sets ground rules to prevent members from inadvertently triggering others' trauma responses.

- **Trustworthiness:** Building and maintaining trust is fundamental. This extends beyond clear communication about treatment; it also involves consistency in actions and follow-through. For instance, if a healthcare provider says they will follow up with a resource, doing so in a timely manner reinforces trust. In practice, this principle ensures that clients are aware of their rights, the confidentiality of their sessions, and that they have a clear understanding of any treatment or intervention before it begins.

- **Choice:** Empowering clients with choice reinforces a sense of control that trauma often strips away. This can be as simple as giving clients the option to choose between different types of therapy modalities or deciding which topics they are ready to explore in sessions. In group settings, participants might vote on which subjects to discuss each week. Additionally, offering choices in smaller decisions, like the type of music played during a session or the choice of appointment times, can significantly enhance a client's sense of autonomy.

- **Collaboration:** This principle is about recognizing the client as an equal partner in their healing journey. It's exemplified when a counselor not only sets goals with a client but also asks for feedback on the therapy process itself. Collaborative approaches might include joint decision-making in community programs, where individuals with lived experience of trauma contribute to the design and evaluation of services that affect them.

- **Empowerment:** A focus on empowerment involves identifying and drawing upon the client's inherent strengths. In practice, this could involve a counselor noticing a client's resilience in facing challenges and reflecting this back to the client. In educational settings, teachers might encourage students who have experienced trauma to lead projects on topics where they feel strong and competent. Empowerment is also about providing opportunities for skill-building, such as a job-training program that helps individuals learn new skills in a supportive, pace-sensitive environment.

By integrating these principles into practice, service providers can create a supportive framework that not only recognizes and responds to the effects of trauma but actively works to counteract its negative impact. This holistic approach is about more than avoiding re-traumatization; it's about fostering an environment where individuals can thrive and regain a sense of control and self-worth in their lives.

### Implementing Trauma-Informed Care:

Incorporating trauma-informed care (TIC) into various service settings is essential for accommodating individuals who have experienced trauma. It requires a concerted effort across all levels of an organization. Here's how to approach this:

1. **Staff Training:**

   - It's imperative that every member of an organization, from the front desk to the back office, understands the fundamentals of TIC. Receptionists, for example, should be trained to use language that is non-triggering when asking for personal information. They might say, "Please let me know any details you feel comfortable sharing with us," as opposed to directly probing personal or potentially triggering information.

   - Maintenance staff could be trained to recognize that sudden loud noises can be unsettling for some individuals and learn to give a heads-up before performing tasks that could cause such disturbances.

2. **Policy Development:**

   - Policies should be crafted to ensure that the procedures of an organization do not inadvertently re-traumatize individuals. For example, a policy might be to always ask for consent before closing the door in a counseling session, providing a sense of control to the individual.

   - A policy could include guidelines for a private space where individuals can take breaks if they feel overwhelmed, ensuring they have a safe place to regroup.

3. **Service Adaptation:**

   - Adapt services to the individual needs of those who have experienced trauma. For instance, a dental office might recognize that lying supine in a chair can be triggering for some individuals. Offering the option to take breaks or sit up periodically during procedures can be helpful.

   - In educational settings, teachers can offer alternative assignments if the subject matter could potentially be triggering, ensuring that students are not forced to engage with material that could harm their emotional state.

4. **Environment:**

   - The physical space of service delivery should convey safety and calm. In a counseling center, this could mean private waiting areas for those who may feel vulnerable in public spaces.

   - In hospitals, offering rooms with adjustable lighting can help individuals who may feel stressed by harsh, fluorescent lights.

   - Even in virtual spaces, such as support hotlines, creating a soothing auditory environment with soft background music during hold times can contribute to a sense of calm.

By integrating TIC principles into all aspects of service provision, organizations can create a supportive environment that acknowledges and respects the needs of individuals with trauma histories. This holistic approach does not just minimize the risk of re-traumatization but actively contributes to the healing process, facilitating a path to recovery that is both compassionate and respectful.

**Examples of Trauma-Informed Care (TIC) in the Context of HIV Stigma**

- **Creating a Non-Judgmental Environment:**

  - A healthcare provider ensures their clinic space is welcoming and free from stigmatizing materials or messages about HIV. They use inclusive language in brochures and posters, emphasizing the dignity and respect of all clients, regardless of their HIV status.

- **Sensitive Communication during Consultations:**

  - During medical consultations, clinicians use person-first language and avoid stigmatizing terms when discussing HIV. For example, they say, "a person living with HIV" instead of "HIV patient," and focus on the individual's overall health and well-being, not just their HIV status.

- **Training Staff on HIV-Related Stigma:**

  - All staff members, including non-medical personnel, receive training on the realities of living with HIV, the impact of stigma, and ways to communicate sensitively and supportively with clients who have experienced stigma.

- **Confidentiality and Privacy:**

  - Ensuring the highest level of confidentiality in handling the medical records and information of clients living with HIV. Staff members are trained to understand the importance of privacy, especially in small communities where the risk of stigma is high.

- **Support Groups and Peer Counseling:**

  - Facilitating support groups or peer counseling sessions where clients living with HIV can share their experiences in a safe and supportive environment. These groups are led by individuals who are also living with HIV, providing a space for shared understanding and empathy.

- **Addressing Mental Health Needs:**

  - Recognizing the mental health impact of HIV-related stigma, clinicians proactively screen for depression, anxiety, and other mental health issues. They provide or refer clients to appropriate mental health services, including counseling and therapy.

- **Culturally Sensitive Care:**

  - Understanding how cultural backgrounds influence perceptions of HIV and stigma. Providers tailor their approach to be culturally sensitive, which may involve working with cultural liaisons or offering materials in different languages.

- **Empowering Clients Through Education:**

  - Providing clients with comprehensive, up-to-date information about HIV, its treatment, and ways to manage stigma. This empowerment through knowledge helps clients advocate for themselves in various settings, including the workplace, family, and healthcare environments.

In each of these examples, the key is to approach clients with empathy and understanding, acknowledging the additional layer of trauma that HIV stigma can bring. By integrating these practices into care, providers create a more supportive and effective environment for clients dealing with the dual challenges of HIV and stigma.

**Conclusion:**

Trauma-Informed Care (TIC) represents a profound transformation in the delivery of healthcare and social services. It transcends traditional techniques, embodying a philosophy that reshapes our interactions and the environments we create for service provision. This approach is centered on building a nurturing and supportive atmosphere where individuals with trauma histories are not just seen but genuinely understood, where their dignity is upheld, and their stories are woven into the fabric of their care and healing journey.

In practical terms, TIC involves small but significant changes in everyday interactions. For example, in a primary care setting, it might involve a doctor using open-ended questions to invite a dialogue about a patient's history, rather than directly probing into potentially sensitive areas. In a mental health context, it could mean therapists offering flexible scheduling to accommodate clients who may find rigid appointment times stressful due to past experiences.

Moreover, TIC emphasizes the physical environment as well. Consider a dental office that has adapted its space to be more trauma-informed – it may have gentle, calming colors on the walls, private spaces for patients who might feel vulnerable, and staff trained to recognize signs of anxiety or distress.

Educational settings also benefit from this approach. A school that practices TIC might have teachers trained to recognize and sensitively respond to signs of trauma in students, such as by offering quiet, safe spaces for children who are overwhelmed, or integrating mindfulness practices into the classroom to help students regulate their emotions.

In social services, TIC can mean case workers taking the time to build trust with clients, recognizing that many have had past experiences where their trust was betrayed. It's about offering choices and giving control back to those who may have felt powerless, allowing them to guide their service experience.

By adopting TIC, service providers across various sectors can profoundly impact the well-being of those with trauma histories. This approach does not just treat symptoms or address immediate needs; it fosters a healing relationship and a path towards empowerment. Ultimately, TIC is about reshaping our societal approach to care – one that is holistic, empathetic, and deeply respectful of the individual journeys of those who have experienced trauma.

## Knowledge Check

Welcome to the Knowledge Check sections! These segments are designed to enhance your understanding and retention of key concepts discussed in our training. Each section presents a series of thought-provoking questions or problems that will challenge your grasp of the material. By engaging with these questions, you'll have the opportunity to reflect on what you've learned, apply your knowledge in practical scenarios, and deepen your comprehension of the subject matter. These checks are a vital part of the learning process, enabling you to consolidate your learning and identify areas where you may need further clarification or study. Let's dive in and explore these concepts further!

1. **Question:** How does Trauma-Informed Care (TIC) differ from traditional care approaches in handling clients who have experienced trauma?

**Answer:** TIC differs from traditional approaches by prioritizing the understanding of a person's life experiences, especially trauma, in their care. In a traditional setting, a healthcare provider might focus solely on treating symptoms or illnesses. In contrast, a TIC approach involves recognizing signs of trauma in a person's behavior or health condition and adjusting the care accordingly. For example, in TIC, a mental health professional would consider a person's traumatic experiences when discussing treatment options, ensuring that therapies do not inadvertently re-traumatize the individual.

2. **Question:** What are some common missteps in interactions that are not trauma-informed, and how can they be rectified?

**Answer:** A common misstep in non-trauma-informed interactions is making assumptions about a person's behavior or condition without considering the potential impact of past trauma. For instance, labeling a person as 'difficult' or 'non-compliant' without understanding their trauma background can be retraumatizing. To rectify this, professionals should approach behavior with curiosity rather than judgment, asking questions like, "What happened to you?" instead of "What's wrong with you?". This shift in perspective helps in providing care that is sensitive to the individual's trauma history.

3. **Question:** How can a trauma-informed approach be applied in an educational setting, particularly for children with trauma histories?

**Answer:** In an educational setting, TIC involves creating a safe and supportive environment for children, especially those with trauma histories. Teachers and staff can be trained to recognize and respond to trauma signs. For example, instead of punishing a child for disruptive behavior, educators can provide a calm, safe space for the child to regulate their emotions. Schools can also implement policies that emphasize emotional support and counseling, and encourage activities that promote resilience and emotional literacy.

4. **Question:** What role does cultural competency play in delivering Trauma-Informed Care?

**Answer:** Cultural competency is crucial in TIC as it ensures care is respectful and relevant to the cultural background of the individual. Different cultures have varied ways of understanding and responding to trauma. A culturally competent TIC provider will be aware of these differences and tailor their approach accordingly. For example, they might incorporate culturally specific healing practices into treatment plans or ensure translation services are available for individuals who are more comfortable discussing traumatic experiences in their native language.

5. **Question:** How can organizations ensure their policies and procedures are trauma-informed?

**Answer:** Organizations can ensure their policies and procedures are trauma-informed by incorporating TIC principles at every level of operation. This might include training all staff in trauma awareness, creating environments that prioritize safety and comfort, and implementing policies that allow flexibility in service provision. For instance, a healthcare clinic might have a policy that allows patients who have experienced trauma to have a support person present during examinations or treatments.

These questions and answers should provide a deeper understanding of TIC and its application across various settings. Using people-first language and examples helps to contextualize TIC principles in real-world situations, enhancing comprehension and long-term retention of these concepts.

## Introduction to Harm Reduction

Harm reduction is a compassionate, evidence-based approach primarily aimed at supporting individuals who use drugs. It's a strategy that acknowledges drug use as a part of our world and works towards minimizing its harmful effects rather than ignoring or condemning them. This method provides vital tools and information, which can be life-saving and conducive to positive change. Grounded in public health principles, harm reduction focuses on prevention, risk reduction, and health promotion. It's about empowering individuals and their families, enabling them to lead lives that are healthy, self-directed, and purposeful. Central to harm reduction is the respect for the experiences and voices of individuals, especially those from underserved communities, in shaping effective strategies and practices.

**Core Principles of Harm Reduction:**

### Non-Judgmental Approach:

- This principle acknowledges that drug use is a reality in our society. For example, instead of condemning a person for using opioids, harm reduction strategies might include providing access to clean needles or overdose prevention drugs like Naloxone. This approach doesn't insist on abstinence or cessation but rather focuses on reducing harm while respecting individual choices.

### Client-Centered Focus:

- Harm reduction puts the needs and experiences of individuals who use drugs at the forefront. It involves them in making decisions about their care, recognizing them as experts in their own lives. An example is a methadone program where individuals who are dependent on opioids are involved in creating their treatment plan, ensuring it fits their unique needs and life circumstances.

### Harm Minimization:

- This principle seeks to reduce the adverse effects associated with drug use. It recognizes that people who use drugs are individuals with unique needs and circumstances.

- Example: Providing clean syringes to prevent HIV and hepatitis C transmission among people who inject drugs. Offering naloxone kits and training to reduce the risk of overdose fatalities.

### Community-Based Strategies:

- This involves working directly with communities, including people who use drugs, their families, and local organizations. It's about understanding and respecting the specific needs and contexts of each community.

- Example: A neighborhood clinic organizes a community meeting to discuss safe drug consumption spaces, where people who use drugs are welcomed to share their thoughts and needs.

**Collaborative Efforts:**

- Collaborating with a wide range of stakeholders ensures that harm reduction strategies are holistic and effective. This means engaging with healthcare providers, law enforcement, policymakers, and, importantly, the people directly affected by these policies.

- Example: A city's health department partners with local police, medical experts, and people who use drugs to create guidelines that prioritize health and safety over criminalization.

**Evidence-Based Practices:**

- Harm reduction strategies should be grounded in scientific research and continuously updated with the latest data and findings.

- Example: Implementing a needle exchange program after studies show it effectively reduces disease transmission without increasing drug use. Regularly reviewing and updating the program based on new research findings to ensure it remains effective and relevant.

**Harm Reduction Strategies:**

Harm reduction strategies aim to minimize the health risks associated with certain behaviors, particularly in the context of substance use. Here are some of the key strategies, explained with examples for better understanding:

**Needle Exchange Programs:**

- **What it is:** These programs provide clean needles and syringes to individuals, reducing the risk of transmitting HIV and hepatitis C.

- **Example:** John, who uses injectable drugs, visits a needle exchange program where he can safely dispose of used needles and obtain clean ones, significantly reducing his risk of contracting or spreading infections.

**Overdose Prevention:**

- **What it is:** This includes access to naloxone (a medication used to reverse opioid overdoses) and training on how to use it.

- **Example:** Emma, a community health worker, carries naloxone and is trained to use it. She can provide immediate help in case of an opioid overdose in her community, potentially saving lives.

**Safer Drug Use Education:**

- **What it is:** Offering information on safer drug use practices, such as using test strips to detect fentanyl in substances.

- **Example:** A local health center conducts workshops teaching how to use fentanyl test strips, helping people like Alex to make informed decisions and reduce the risk of accidental overdose.

**HIV and Hepatitis C Testing and Treatment:**

- **What it is:** Facilitating testing and treatment services to manage and curb the spread of these diseases.

- **Example:** Sarah, who is at risk, visits a clinic where she gets tested for HIV and Hepatitis C. Upon testing positive, she is immediately linked to treatment services.

**Mental Health and Substance Use Disorder Treatment:**

- **What it is:** Providing treatment options that address the underlying mental health issues related to drug use.

- **Example:** After struggling with anxiety and substance use, Mike finds a treatment center that helps him with both his mental health and substance use disorder, leading to a healthier lifestyle.

**Support for Housing and Employment:**

- **What it is:** Assistance programs aimed at stabilizing individuals' lives by helping them find housing and employment.

- **Example:** Lisa, recovering from substance dependence, gets help from a program that assists her in finding a job and stable housing, greatly contributing to her rehabilitation and reintegration into society.

By understanding and implementing these harm reduction strategies, communities and individuals can work towards safer practices, better health outcomes, and an overall reduction in the harms associated with substance use.

**Implementation in Practice:**

This training is designed as a practical guide to help individuals, organizations, and communities comprehend and apply harm reduction principles effectively. It's crucial to tailor these principles to fit local contexts, ensuring that they are not only relevant and effective but also cater to the specific needs and circumstances of individuals.

For example, in a community where there's a high incidence of opioid use, a local health center might implement harm reduction strategies such as providing access to clean needles and offering naloxone training to reduce the risk of overdoses. Similarly, in a school setting, educators could incorporate harm reduction education into their curriculum, focusing on safe practices and support resources for students who might be experimenting with substances.

**Conclusion:**

Harm reduction plays an essential role in addressing substance use disorders and improving the well-being of people who use drugs. By embedding harm reduction strategies into our policies, programs, and day-to-day practices, we contribute significantly to minimizing the negative health and social impacts of drug use. More importantly, we offer support to people in leading healthier and more self-directed lives.

For instance, by providing safe consumption spaces, we not only reduce the risks associated with substance use but also create opportunities for individuals to access healthcare, counseling, and support services. In educational settings, adopting harm reduction approaches means moving beyond traditional "just say no" messages to provide young people with factual, non-judgmental information about substances, fostering an environment where they feel safe to seek help if needed.

Ultimately, harm reduction is about respecting and supporting the choices of individuals while providing them with the tools and resources to reduce potential harm, thereby embracing a compassionate and person-centered approach to health and well-being.

## Knowledge Check

Welcome to the Knowledge Check sections! These segments are designed to enhance your understanding and retention of key concepts discussed in our training. Each section presents a series of thought-provoking questions or problems that will challenge your grasp of the material. By engaging with these questions, you'll have the opportunity to reflect on what you've learned, apply your knowledge in practical scenarios, and deepen your comprehension of the subject matter. These checks are a vital part of the learning process, enabling you to consolidate your learning and identify areas where you may need further clarification or study. Let's dive in and explore these concepts further!

**Question:** How does harm reduction differ from other substance use treatment approaches, and why is it important in public health?

**Answer:** Harm reduction differs from traditional substance use treatment approaches in its focus on minimizing the negative consequences of drug use rather than solely on eliminating or reducing drug use itself. This approach is important in public health because it recognizes the complexities of drug use and prioritizes the health and safety of individuals. For example, needle exchange programs reduce the risk of transmitting HIV and Hepatitis C among people who inject drugs, without necessarily requiring them to stop using drugs immediately. This approach is vital as it meets people where they are in their journey, offering support and resources that can lead to healthier outcomes, even if they're not ready or able to cease substance use.

**Question:** What are some common harm reduction strategies, and how do they benefit individuals who use drugs?

**Answer:** Common harm reduction strategies include needle exchange programs, providing safe consumption spaces, offering naloxone to reverse opioid overdoses, and education on safer drug use practices. These strategies benefit individuals by reducing the immediate health risks associated with drug use, such as infections from sharing needles or overdosing. For instance, safe consumption spaces not only provide a safer environment for drug use but also offer access to healthcare and social services, creating pathways for individuals to seek further treatment and support.

**Question:** How can harm reduction strategies be effectively communicated to communities that may have a negative perception of drug use?

**Answer:** Effectively communicating harm reduction strategies to communities with negative perceptions of drug use involves focusing on public health benefits, cost-effectiveness, and community safety. It's crucial to use empathetic and non-stigmatizing language that emphasizes the humanity and dignity of individuals who use drugs. For example, highlighting how needle exchange programs have been effective in reducing the spread of infectious diseases in a community can shift the perspective from moral judgment to public health necessity. Additionally, sharing success stories and statistics on how harm reduction strategies have positively impacted other communities can help in building acceptance and support.

**Question:** What role do social determinants of health play in harm reduction, and how can they be addressed in harm reduction strategies?

**Answer:** Social determinants of health, such as poverty, lack of access to healthcare, education, and stable housing, significantly impact substance use and the effectiveness of harm reduction strategies. Addressing these factors is crucial in harm reduction as they often underlie the reasons for substance use and can hinder access to harm reduction services. Strategies like integrating substance use services with other social services, offering mobile health units in underserved areas, and advocating for policies that address poverty and homelessness can be effective. For example, providing housing-first initiatives for homeless individuals who use drugs can create a stable environment where they can more effectively engage in harm reduction and other health services.

**Question:** What are some challenges in implementing harm reduction policies, and how can they be overcome?

**Answer:** Challenges in implementing harm reduction policies include stigma, lack of funding, political opposition, and community resistance. Overcoming these challenges involves advocacy, education, and building coalitions with stakeholders, including healthcare providers, law enforcement, and community groups. For example, engaging community leaders and stakeholders in open dialogues about the benefits of harm reduction and addressing their concerns can build support. Securing funding may involve demonstrating the cost-effectiveness of harm reduction in reducing healthcare expenses long-term. Overcoming stigma requires consistent public education campaigns that humanize people who use drugs and highlight the public health benefits of harm reduction.

This section aims to provide guidance on the use of person-first language, particularly in the context of HIV and other health conditions. Person-first language is essential in respectful and empathetic communication, emphasizing the individuality of each person over their medical condition.

**What is Person-First Language?**

Person-first language is a respectful and compassionate way of communicating that acknowledges a person's identity first, rather than leading with their health condition. For instance, instead of saying "an HIV patient," which defines a person by their condition, we say "a person living with HIV." This subtle yet powerful shift in language emphasizes the person's humanity and places the condition as only one aspect of their multifaceted life.

**Why Person-First Language Matters:**

- **Promotes Dignity:** It asserts that a person is not solely defined by their condition. For example, saying "a person with diabetes" instead of "a diabetic" prevents reducing the individual's identity to their medical state.

- **Encourages Empathy:** It reminds us that everyone has unique experiences and challenges. When we speak of "a child with asthma" rather than "an asthmatic child," we're considering the child's experiences and challenges with empathy.

- **Reduces Stigma:** By not leading with the condition, we help combat the stigma that can be associated with medical diagnoses. Referring to "a person experiencing addiction" rather than "an addict" can help shift perceptions and reduce judgment.

**Examples of Person-First Language:**

| Non-Person-First Term | Person-First Term | Why It's Important |
| --- | --- | --- |
| HIV patient | Person living with HIV | Acknowledges that the person has a life beyond their HIV status. |
| Diabetic | Person with diabetes | Emphasizes that having diabetes is just one aspect of the person. |
| Disabled person | Person with a disability | Puts the person before the disability, noting it does not define them. |
| Addict | Person with a substance use disorder | Recognizes the medical condition as a disorder that can be treated. |

**Implementing Person-First Language:**

- **In Healthcare Settings:** Medical professionals can model person-first language, setting a standard of respect and care in treatment settings.

- **In the Workplace:** Employers and coworkers using person-first language can foster an inclusive and supportive environment.

- **In Grant Writing and Communication:** Journalists, writers, and public speakers can use person-first language to influence public perception and discourse.

- **In Education:** Teachers and educational materials that use person-first language can shape understanding from a young age.

Person-first language is more than a linguistic preference; it's a reflection of our values and attitudes towards all individuals, particularly those living with health conditions like HIV. By placing the person before the condition, we affirm their dignity, encourage empathy, and take a stand against stigma. It's a practice that, when adopted widely, has the power to transform societal attitudes and improve the lives of many.

**Examples and Application in Different Contexts:**

### HIV/AIDS:

- Use "a person living with HIV" rather than "an HIV patient."

- Use "a person affected by AIDS" instead of "an AIDS victim."

- **Example Context:** In a healthcare setting, when discussing protocols, one might say, "People living with HIV will be offered the latest antiretroviral treatments" instead of referring to them as "HIV patients."

### Mental Health Conditions:

- Say "a person with schizophrenia" instead of "a schizophrenic."

- Use "a person with bipolar disorder" rather than "a bipolar."

- **Example Context:** In therapeutic discussions, you might frame it as, "We're looking at support strategies for people experiencing schizophrenia," rather than labeling them "schizophrenics."

### Neurodiversity:

- Refer to "a person with autism" instead of "an autistic person."

- Say "a person with dyslexia" rather than "a dyslexic."

- **Example Context:** An educator might say, "We provide specialized reading programs for students with autism" rather than "autistic students."

### Chronic Conditions:

- Use "a person with diabetes" instead of "a diabetic."

- Say "a person with epilepsy" rather than "an epileptic."

- **Example Context:** A public health announcement might include, "We offer resources for people with epilepsy to manage their condition" instead of referring to them as "epileptics."

**Physical Disabilities:**

- Prefer "a person with a disability" over "a disabled person."

- Use "a person who uses a wheelchair" rather than "a wheelchair-bound person."

- **Example Context:** In accessibility planning, one might read, "The building's design includes features for persons with disabilities, like ramps for people who use wheelchairs," avoiding the term "wheelchair-bound."

Using person-first language conveys respect and emphasizes the person, not the condition. It's a key component in communication that fosters dignity and counters stigma.

**Conclusion:**

Embracing person-first language in our communication is a vital move towards cultivating a society that is more respectful, inclusive, and empathetic. This approach is especially pivotal in healthcare and social service settings, where the choice of language can profoundly affect the mental and emotional well-being of individuals. Person-first language places the emphasis on the individual rather than the condition, thereby respecting and acknowledging the dignity and uniqueness of each person. Such language fosters a more compassionate and less stigmatizing atmosphere. It's crucial to recognize that our words, both spoken and written, have the power to shape perceptions and influence how individuals are treated and viewed within society. This mindful approach to communication is a key step in promoting dignity and understanding for everyone.

## Knowledge Check

Welcome to the Knowledge Check sections! These segments are designed to enhance your understanding and retention of key concepts discussed in our training. Each section presents a series of thought-provoking questions or problems that will challenge your grasp of the material. By engaging with these questions, you'll have the opportunity to reflect on what you've learned, apply your knowledge in practical scenarios, and deepen your comprehension of the subject matter. These checks are a vital part of the learning process, enabling you to consolidate your learning and identify areas where you may need further clarification or study. Let's dive in and explore these concepts further!

**Question: What is the potential impact of not using person-first language when discussing individuals with chronic diseases in a healthcare setting?**

**Answer:** Not using person-first language in a healthcare setting can have a significant negative impact on individuals with chronic diseases. It can contribute to a stigmatizing environment where the condition defines the individual, rather than seeing them as a multifaceted person who has an illness. For example, referring to someone as a "diabetic" focuses solely on their disease, whereas saying "person with diabetes" recognizes them as an individual first. The former can lead to feelings of being labeled, reduced to an illness, and experiencing discrimination, which can impact their self-esteem, treatment adherence, and quality of care. Person-first language promotes dignity, respect, and empathy, essential for holistic care.

**Question: How might person-first language improve the dynamics of a support group for mental health?**

**Answer:** In a support group setting, using person-first language helps to create a more supportive, respectful, and empowering environment. It shifts the focus from the mental health condition to the individual's experiences, strengths, and identity. For instance, saying "individuals with bipolar disorder" rather than "bipolar patients" emphasizes the person's humanity and not just their mental health status. This can encourage group members to share their experiences and strategies for coping, reinforcing the idea that they have control over their lives, rather than being controlled by their condition. It can also enhance mutual understanding and reduce prejudice, leading to a stronger, more connected support network.

**Question: How can person-first language be problematic, and what's an alternative inclusive language approach?**

**Answer:** Person-first language, while well-intentioned, can sometimes be problematic if it unintentionally emphasizes the condition by constantly drawing attention to it. Some individuals may prefer identity-first language, which acknowledges that the condition is an integral part of their identity and does not necessarily need to be separated. For example, many in the Deaf community prefer "Deaf person" over "person with deafness" because deafness is seen as a cultural identity rather than a condition to be mitigated. The best approach is to ask individuals how they prefer to be addressed and to respect personal and community language preferences. It's about being adaptable and person-centered in our language choices.

**Question: If a journalist is writing an article about a person who has been homeless, how should they apply person-first language to communicate respectfully?**

**Answer:** A journalist should apply person-first language by separating the condition or situation from the individual. Instead of labeling someone as "a homeless person," which defines them by their housing status, they should say "a person experiencing homelessness." This phrasing acknowledges that homelessness is a temporary and surmountable situation, not a defining characteristic. It helps to maintain the subject's dignity and promotes the understanding that homelessness is a complex issue that could be faced by anyone, rather than a personal failing.

**Question: In educational settings, how can person-first language affect the integration of students with disabilities?**

**Answer:** Using person-first language in educational settings can greatly impact the inclusion and integration of students with disabilities. By referring to "students with disabilities" rather than "disabled students," educators and peers are reminded that the students are not defined by their disabilities. This can influence how educational strategies are implemented, ensuring that they are tailored to meet the needs of each student as an individual. It can also affect peer interactions, promoting a more inclusive environment where students are seen for their abilities rather than their limitations. For example, saying "student with autism" instead of "autistic student" places the student first, which can lead to more emphasis on their individual learning style, interests, and talents. This approach fosters a supportive and empowering environment for all students.

## Harm Reduction Through Status Neutral HIV Prevention and Care

This section is dedicated to offering a comprehensive exploration of the Status Neutral approach to HIV Prevention and Care. This holistic and inclusive strategy represents a paradigm shift in HIV-related healthcare, emphasizing equal and comprehensive care for every individual. Designed to transcend the boundaries of HIV status, this approach ensures that all individuals, whether living with HIV or seeking preventive measures, receive equitable and uninterrupted access to healthcare services. By embracing this approach, we aim to foster an environment where healthcare equity is not just an ideal, but a practical reality.

**Understanding Status Neutrality**

### What is Status Neutral HIV Prevention and Care?

- This is a comprehensive approach that ensures high-quality HIV prevention and care for everyone. It integrates and balances the needs of those living with HIV and those seeking prevention services.

- Example: In a status neutral system, a person seeking an HIV test is also provided with information on both HIV treatment options and preventive measures like Pre-Exposure Prophylaxis (PrEP), regardless of their test result.

### Why Embrace Status Neutrality?

**Achieving Optimal Health and Well-being:** The goal is to provide every individual impacted by HIV the best possible health outcomes, through continuous and comprehensive care.

- Example: A person diagnosed with HIV is immediately linked to antiretroviral therapy (ART) and also provided with mental health support and counseling services, addressing both medical and psychosocial needs.

**Destigmatizing HIV Treatment and Prevention:** By normalizing HIV-related services, status neutrality helps to break down the stigma associated with HIV, encouraging more people to seek testing and care.

- Example: Public health campaigns that promote HIV testing as a routine part of healthcare, similar to regular blood pressure or cholesterol checks, help normalize the process and reduce stigma.

**Unified Access to Services:** It streamlines access to healthcare and social services, making it easier for individuals to receive the care they need.

- Example: A community health center offering a range of services from HIV testing and treatment to mental health care and nutritional support under one roof simplifies access and reduces barriers to care.

**Whole Person Approach:**

- This involves acknowledging and addressing the unique needs and circumstances of each individual.

- For example, a person living with HIV might also need mental health support or assistance with transportation to healthcare appointments. A status neutral approach ensures these needs are met alongside HIV treatment.

**Addressing Social and Structural Barriers:**

- This component focuses on identifying and overcoming obstacles to accessing HIV prevention and care.

- For instance, if individuals face difficulty accessing Pre-exposure Prophylaxis (PrEP) due to lack of insurance, a status neutral approach might involve connecting them to programs that provide PrEP at a reduced cost or for free.

**Comprehensive Support and Care:**

- Support extends beyond medical treatment to include factors like housing stability, mental health, and food security.

- An example would be a clinic that not only offers Antiretroviral Therapy (ART) but also connects clients to housing services or mental health counseling, addressing the holistic needs of the individual.

**Entry Point to Care:**

- The HIV test is considered the initial engagement point, where assessment and care begin.

- Regardless of whether a person tests positive or negative, their needs are assessed at this stage. For example, someone testing negative might be guided towards preventive measures like PrEP, while someone testing positive immediately receives information about ART.

**Modifying Care Continuum:**

- This involves transitioning from a disease-centric model to a holistic, needs-based approach.

- For example, rather than following a standard protocol for all HIV-positive individuals, the care plan is tailored to each person's unique health profile and life situation.

**Community Engagement:**

- This aspect emphasizes expanding the availability and accessibility of services for the entire community.

- An example could include community outreach programs that offer HIV education and testing in various settings, such as schools, workplaces, or local events, ensuring that all community members have access to essential services.

By incorporating these components, the status neutral approach ensures that every individual receives personalized, comprehensive care and support, significantly contributing to better health outcomes and reduced HIV-related stigma.

## Implementing Status Neutral Approach

## In Practice:

### Integration into Healthcare Systems:

- Health departments are encouraged to adopt status neutral models in their healthcare strategies. This involves treating all individuals with the same level of care and attention, regardless of their HIV status.

- Example: A clinic might offer both HIV testing and general health screenings in the same visit, ensuring that all patients receive comprehensive care.

### Universal HIV Testing:

- Facilitate HIV testing for everyone, regardless of perceived risk, to ensure early detection and intervention.

- Example: Implementing routine HIV testing in all healthcare settings, from general practitioners to emergency departments, to normalize and destigmatize the process.

### Personalized Prevention and Treatment:

- Provide tailored prevention and treatment options based on individual needs, preferences, and circumstances.

- Example: Offering Pre-Exposure Prophylaxis (PrEP) to individuals at high risk of HIV alongside other preventive healthcare measures.

### Comprehensive Support Services:

- Connect individuals to a range of services and support mechanisms that cater to their holistic needs, such as mental health counseling, social services, and community support groups.

- Example: Referring a patient diagnosed with HIV to both medical treatment and a mental health professional for comprehensive care.

## Benefits:

### Reduction in New HIV Infections:

- By providing universal testing and immediate access to prevention and treatment, the spread of HIV can be significantly reduced.

- Example: In areas where status neutral approaches have been implemented, such as San Francisco, a notable decrease in new HIV infections has been observed.

**Improved Access to Care:**

- The status neutral approach eliminates barriers to accessing care, ensuring that all individuals, regardless of their HIV status, can receive the services they need.

- Example: A person testing negative for HIV can readily access preventive services, while someone testing positive is immediately linked to treatment programs.

**Decreased HIV-Related Stigma:**

- By normalizing HIV testing and treatment as part of general healthcare, the stigma associated with HIV can be significantly reduced.

- Example: Regular HIV testing as part of routine health check-ups can help to normalize the condition, reducing fear and misinformation.

In summary, implementing a status neutral approach in healthcare not only aids in effective HIV management but also fosters an inclusive, non-discriminatory healthcare environment. This approach can lead to better health outcomes for individuals and communities by reducing new infections, improving access to care, and decreasing stigma related to HIV.

**Conclusion**

Adopting a Status Neutral approach in HIV prevention and care represents a crucial advancement in delivering personalized and effective healthcare. This approach is centered on respecting and addressing the unique needs and circumstances of each individual, contributing significantly to the reduction of HIV transmission and improving the overall health and well-being of those impacted by HIV. By considering the whole person, rather than focusing solely on their HIV status, this method promotes a more inclusive and equitable healthcare system. Such an approach not only aids in bridging healthcare disparities but also plays a vital role in dismantling the stigma associated with HIV. Embracing Status Neutral care thus marks a pivotal move towards achieving health equity, where every individual receives high-quality, comprehensive care irrespective of their HIV status, paving the way for a healthier, more inclusive society.

## Knowledge Check

Welcome to the Knowledge Check sections! These segments are designed to enhance your understanding and retention of key concepts discussed in our training. Each section presents a series of thought-provoking questions or problems that will challenge your grasp of the material. By engaging with these questions, you'll have the opportunity to reflect on what you've learned, apply your knowledge in practical scenarios, and deepen your comprehension of the subject matter. These checks are a vital part of the learning process, enabling you to consolidate your learning and identify areas where you may need further clarification or study. Let's dive in and explore these concepts further!

1. **Question:** How does the status neutral approach to HIV prevention and care contribute to reducing the stigma associated with HIV testing and treatment? Provide an example.

**Answer:** The status neutral approach integrates HIV prevention and care into general healthcare, making HIV-related services a routine part of medical care rather than an exceptional or stigmatized activity. This normalizes both the discussion and treatment of HIV, reducing the fear and shame often associated with the virus. For example, when HIV testing is offered as a standard part of a health check-up, just like blood pressure or cholesterol tests, it becomes a normal healthcare practice rather than an indicator of risk or moral judgment. This normalization can significantly reduce the stigma and discrimination often faced by individuals living with or at risk of HIV.

2. **Question:** What challenges might health departments face in implementing a status neutral approach, and how can they be addressed?

**Answer:** Challenges in implementing a status neutral approach may include resource constraints, lack of awareness or training among healthcare providers, and resistance from communities due to existing stigmas. Addressing these challenges involves securing funding for comprehensive services, providing thorough training for healthcare professionals in status neutral practices, and conducting community outreach and education to shift public perception and understanding of HIV. An example of addressing these challenges would be a health department organizing workshops for healthcare providers to educate them about the status neutral approach and its benefits, alongside community awareness programs to inform the public about the new model of care.

3. **Question:** How does the status neutral approach ensure personalized and comprehensive care for individuals regardless of their HIV status?

**Answer:** The status neutral approach focuses on the individual needs of each person rather than solely their HIV status. It offers tailored services, including prevention, treatment, and support, based on a person's unique health profile, lifestyle, and social circumstances. For instance, a person who tests negative for HIV might receive information and access to preventive measures like PrEP, while someone who tests positive is provided with immediate antiretroviral therapy and linked to support services like mental health counseling. This personalized care ensures that each person receives the most appropriate and effective services for their specific situation.

4. **Question:** In what ways can the status neutral approach to HIV prevention and care promote health equity?

**Answer:** The status neutral approach promotes health equity by ensuring that all individuals have equal access to HIV prevention and care services, regardless of their status, background, or circumstances. By removing barriers to care and addressing the needs of all community members, this approach helps to reduce health disparities, especially among marginalized groups who are often disproportionately affected by HIV. An example would be a community health center providing both HIV treatment for positive individuals and preventive services like PrEP and education for at-risk populations, ensuring that everyone, irrespective of their socio-economic or health status, receives the care they need.

These questions aim to deepen your understanding of the Harm Reduction Through Status Neutral approach in HIV care, encouraging critical thinking and application of the approach in diverse scenarios.

Sexual health is a vital aspect of overall health and wellness. This section is dedicated to deepening the understanding and advancement of sexual health, with a special emphasis on HIV prevention and care. It covers a comprehensive array of topics, including safer sex practices, which are essential for reducing the risk of HIV transmission and other sexually transmitted infections. Additionally, the section explores the significant influence of mental health on sexual well-being, acknowledging the interconnection between psychological health and sexual health. By addressing these topics, the aim is to promote a holistic approach to sexual health, recognizing its integral role in maintaining a healthy and fulfilling life.

**Safer Sex Practices**

Safer sex practices play a crucial role in minimizing the risk of HIV transmission and other sexually transmitted infections (STIs).

**Condom Use:**

- Correct and consistent use of condoms is one of the most effective ways to prevent HIV and STI transmission during sexual activity.

- **Example:** Educate on the importance of wearing condoms for the entire duration of sexual intercourse. This includes understanding how to properly open a condom package to avoid tearing, checking the expiry date, and ensuring the condom is right-side-out before rolling it on. Highlight the need to choose the right size and type of condom for both comfort and effectiveness. For instance, latex condoms are widely recommended for protection against HIV and STIs, but for individuals with latex allergies, polyurethane or polyisoprene condoms are suitable alternatives.

**Regular Testing:**

- Frequent testing for HIV and other STIs is vital for early detection and treatment, which is beneficial both for the individual's health and for preventing transmission to others.

- **Example:** Implementing regular health check-up campaigns or providing information on where and how to get tested can encourage this practice. For instance, many community health centers and clinics offer free or low-cost testing services for HIV and other STIs.

**Pre-exposure Prophylaxis (PrEP):**

**Understanding PrEP:**

- PrEP is a preventative measure for individuals who do not have HIV but are at substantial risk of acquiring it. This daily medication acts as a safeguard against HIV infection.

- Mechanism: PrEP contains medications that block key pathways that HIV uses to establish an infection. If exposed to HIV, these medications stop the virus from taking hold and spreading in the body.

**Examples and Eligibility:**

- **Individuals with an HIV-Positive Partner:** For instance, a person in a relationship with an HIV-positive partner can use PrEP as a proactive measure to reduce their risk of contracting HIV, even if their partner is receiving antiretroviral therapy.

- **High Risk of Exposure:** This includes people who might not consistently use condoms during sex with partners of unknown HIV status, particularly those in areas with high rates of HIV. Healthcare workers with occupational exposure risks (e.g., needlestick injuries) may also be considered for PrEP.

- **Substance Users:** Individuals who inject drugs and share needles or other injection equipment are at increased risk. PrEP can be a part of a comprehensive harm-reduction strategy for these individuals.

- **We all have a status:** We all have health statuses, and it's important to recognize that some individuals may not know their own or their sexual partners' HIV status. Likewise, there are people who may be unaware of their own health conditions, such as cancer, STIs, TB, or HIV, among others. Acknowledging and respecting each person's unique health circumstances is essential in fostering informed health choices and compassionate care.

**Post-exposure Prophylaxis (PEP):**

Post-exposure Prophylaxis, known as PEP, is a preventive medical treatment initiated after a potential exposure to HIV. This treatment comprises medications that reduce the likelihood of the virus establishing itself in the body.

- Example: If an individual experiences an accidental needlestick injury at work, it is critical for them to start PEP within 72 hours of the potential exposure. The window is crucial as the efficacy of PEP decreases significantly after this period. Once started, the individual would continue the treatment for a full 28-day course.

**Sexual Health and Aging:**

As individuals age, their sexual health needs and challenges can undergo significant changes. It's important to recognize and address these evolving aspects with sensitivity and understanding.

**Adapting to Changing Needs:**

- **Physical Changes:** With age, both men and women experience physical changes that can affect sexual health. For instance, men may encounter issues like erectile dysfunction, which can be both a physical and psychological concern. Meanwhile, women going through menopause might experience vaginal dryness or hormonal fluctuations that impact their sexual experience.

- **Psychological Aspects:** Aging can also bring about psychological changes impacting sexual health. Concerns about body image, self-esteem, or the loss of a partner can affect sexual desire and needs.

- **Health Conditions and Medications:** The onset of chronic health conditions and the use of various medications can have side effects that impact sexual function and desire. It's important to understand how conditions like diabetes or heart disease, and their corresponding treatments, can influence sexual health.

**Importance of Regular Sexual Health Check-ups:**

- **Proactive Health Management:** For older adults, regular sexual health check-ups are crucial. These appointments provide an opportunity to discuss and manage conditions like erectile dysfunction or hormonal changes due to menopause.

- **Screening for Health Issues:** These check-ups also serve as a platform for healthcare providers to screen for other health issues that might affect sexual health, such as prostate health in men or cervical health in women.

- **Open Communication:** Regular discussions with healthcare providers encourage open communication about sexual health, helping to destigmatize these conversations and address issues proactively.

**Navigating Common Issues:**

- **Erectile Dysfunction:** This is a common issue where older men might face challenges in achieving or maintaining an erection. It can stem from both physical health issues, like heart disease or diabetes, and psychological factors such as anxiety or depression.

- **Menopause and Sexual Health:** Women experiencing menopause may face challenges like decreased libido or discomfort during sex due to vaginal dryness. Hormone therapy and other treatments can be effective in managing these symptoms.

As individuals age, their approach to sexual health needs to adapt to their changing bodies and circumstances. Regular check-ups, open communication with healthcare providers, and an understanding of how aging can impact sexual health are key to maintaining sexual well-being in later life.

**Sexual Health and Mental Health:**

Sexual health and mental health are deeply interconnected, with each significantly impacting the other. It's essential to recognize and address mental health issues to maintain a healthy sexual life.

- **Interlinked Aspects:**
    - Mental health influences various aspects of sexual health. For example, an individual's emotional and psychological well-being can directly affect their sexual desire, experience, and performance.

- Likewise, sexual health issues can lead to or exacerbate mental health problems. The stress or anxiety surrounding sexual health can impact overall mental well-being.

**Example of the Connection:**

- Consider a person experiencing depression. This mental health condition can lead to a decreased interest in sexual activity, often impacting their sexual desire and performance. The lack of desire or difficulty in sexual performance can then further contribute to feelings of low self-esteem or worsen the depression, creating a cyclical impact.

- On the other hand, anxiety disorders can also play a significant role. For instance, a person with performance anxiety may experience significant stress and worry about sexual encounters, which can lead to difficulties in sexual performance, such as erectile dysfunction in men or reduced lubrication in women. This can create a cycle of anxiety and sexual difficulties that further impact mental health.

**The Importance of Seeking Support:**

- It's crucial for individuals facing such challenges to seek mental health support. Addressing the underlying mental health issues can often alleviate some of the sexual health problems.

- Therapy, counseling, or medication, as advised by healthcare professionals, can be beneficial. Additionally, open communication with partners and seeking support from sexual health experts can also play a vital role in managing these interconnected aspects of health.

Understanding the intricate link between sexual and mental health is key to holistic well-being. Addressing mental health issues not only improves sexual health but also enhances overall quality of life.

**Sexual Health and Substance Use:**

In addressing sexual health, it's crucial to consider the impact of substance use on decision-making and risk-taking behaviors. This approach emphasizes understanding the individual's experiences and choices while offering support and information.

- **Understanding the Risks Associated with Substance Use:**
  The use of substances can heighten the chance of impulsive risk taking behaviors. This risk is not solely due to the direct effects of the substances themselves but also because of how they can alter judgment and decision-making processes.

Example: Consider a scenario where an individual might engage in substance use at a social gathering. Under the influence of these substances, their ability to make informed and safe decisions regarding sexual activity may be compromised. This impairment can lead to engaging in unprotected sex, which significantly increases the risk of HIV transmission.

- **Discussion and Harm Reduction Strategies:**
  An essential part of this conversation involves discussing strategies for harm reduction. These strategies are not about judgment or forcing change but about providing information and support to help individuals make safer choices.

Example: This could include educating about the use of protection during sexual activities, even when under the influence of substances. It also involves providing information on resources such as local clinics for regular sexual health check-ups, or places where they can receive counseling and support for substance use issues.

A person-first approach to sexual health and substance use focuses on empowering individuals with information and support. By understanding the unique challenges posed by substance use, individuals can be better equipped to make informed decisions that protect their health and well-being.

**Sexual Health in Relationships:**

**Communication and Consent in Sexual Health:**

- Prioritizing open and honest communication about sexual health in relationships is crucial. It's important for individuals to engage in discussions with their partners about their sexual health, preferences, and boundaries to ensure mutual understanding and respect.

- **Example:** Consider a scenario where two individuals are in a new relationship. Before becoming intimate, they sit down to have a candid conversation about their sexual health histories. They discuss when they were last tested for sexually transmitted infections (STIs) and agree to get tested together as a proactive step. Additionally, they talk about their preferences regarding contraceptive methods and mutually decide to use condoms to ensure safer sex practices.

**Practicing Consensual, Safer Sex:**

- Consent is a foundational aspect of any healthy sexual relationship. It's essential for all individuals involved to freely and enthusiastically agree to any sexual activity. Additionally, incorporating safer sex practices like the use of condoms or dental dams can significantly reduce the risk of STI transmission and unplanned pregnancies.

- **Example:** Picture a scenario where a couple has been dating for a while. One partner initiates a conversation about potentially stopping the use of condoms, suggesting an alternative form of birth control. They openly discuss their comfort levels, concerns, and the need for recent STI tests. After a thorough and respectful discussion, they reach a mutual decision that honors both of their needs and comfort levels.

By emphasizing person-first language and real-life examples, this text underlines the importance of communication, consent, and safer sex practices in relationships. It encourages individuals to approach discussions about sexual health with empathy, respect, and a commitment to mutual well-being.

**Sexual Health Across Gender Identities:**

- **Prioritizing Inclusivity in Care:** Recognizing and respecting the unique sexual health needs of individuals with diverse gender identities is essential. This approach ensures that everyone receives appropriate and effective health care, tailored to their specific requirements.

    - Example: An individual who identifies as transgender may have specific health needs related to hormone therapy or surgery. Gender-affirmative care in this context involves discussing these unique needs and providing relevant sexual health services. It's crucial for healthcare providers to create a safe and welcoming environment, where patients feel comfortable discussing their gender identity and sexual health concerns.

- **Addressing Specific Needs of Transgender and Non-binary Individuals:** People who are transgender or non-binary often face unique sexual health challenges and risks. Providing care that acknowledges and addresses these specific needs is key to effective treatment and support.

    - Example: A transgender man may require cervical cancer screening if he has not undergone a hysterectomy, a fact that might not be immediately obvious. Healthcare providers should be aware of such nuances and proactively offer relevant screenings and preventive care. Similarly, a non-binary individual might seek advice on safe sex practices that are relevant to their specific anatomy and sexual activities.

Sexual health care that is sensitive to and inclusive of diverse gender identities is not just about recognizing different needs but also about actively facilitating an environment where all individuals feel seen, respected, and cared for. This approach leads to better health outcomes and a more positive healthcare experience for everyone.


**Understanding U=U (Undetectable = Untransmittable):**

U=U, or "Undetectable equals Untransmittable," is a crucial concept in HIV education, particularly for individuals living with HIV. It emphasizes the fact that when a person living with HIV maintains an undetectable viral load through effective treatment, they cannot transmit the virus through sexual contact.

**Significance for Individuals Living with HIV:**

- For people living with HIV, achieving and maintaining an undetectable viral load is not only beneficial for their own health but also crucial in preventing HIV transmission to sexual partners.

- Understanding U=U can significantly reduce the stigma associated with HIV, as it underscores that being on effective treatment eliminates the risk of sexual transmission.

**Real-World Examples:**

- Consider the story of Alex, a person living with HIV who, through consistent treatment, has maintained an undetectable viral load for several years. Alex leads a fulfilling sexual life with their partner, who is HIV-negative. This scenario highlights how understanding and applying the

U=U principle can positively impact personal relationships and reduce anxiety about transmission.

- Another example is Jordan, who was diagnosed with HIV five years ago. Through regular treatment and healthcare support, Jordan has achieved an undetectable viral load, allowing them to focus on their career and personal aspirations without the constant fear of transmitting the virus to others.

By embracing the U=U message, individuals living with HIV can experience a greater sense of freedom and normalcy in their relationships and daily life. This understanding is a powerful tool in combating the stigma surrounding HIV and enhancing the quality of life for those affected by the virus.

In conclusion, it is crucial to address topics related to sexual health to effectively reduce the spread of HIV and other sexually transmitted infections (STIs). By delivering comprehensive education and fostering open discussions about sexual health, we can enhance understanding and create an inclusive and supportive environment. This approach is beneficial for everyone, irrespective of their HIV status or sexual orientation.

Embracing person-first language, it's essential to recognize each individual's unique experiences and needs in the realm of sexual health. Through informed and empathetic conversations, we can build a community that is better equipped to support sexual health and well-being for all.

## Knowledge Check

Welcome to the Knowledge Check sections! These segments are designed to enhance your understanding and retention of key concepts discussed in our training. Each section presents a series of thought-provoking questions or problems that will challenge your grasp of the material. By engaging with these questions, you'll have the opportunity to reflect on what you've learned, apply your knowledge in practical scenarios, and deepen your comprehension of the subject matter. These checks are a vital part of the learning process, enabling you to consolidate your learning and identify areas where you may need further clarification or study. Let's dive in and explore these concepts further!

**Question:** What are the implications of undiagnosed sexually transmitted infections (STIs) on an individual's overall health, and how can healthcare systems encourage more people to get tested?

**Answer:** Undiagnosed STIs can lead to a range of serious health issues, including infertility, chronic pain, or increased risk of transmission. They can also have asymptomatic periods, making individuals unaware they're affected and inadvertently transmitting the infection to others. To encourage testing, healthcare systems can implement confidential, accessible, and non-stigmatizing services. For instance, offering STI testing as a routine part of medical care, regardless of whether a person shows symptoms, and providing clear, non-judgmental information about the importance of regular testing can increase engagement. Educational campaigns that use relatable scenarios, like a person considering STI testing after a new sexual partnership, can also demystify the process and highlight its importance.

**Question 2:**
How does stigma surrounding HIV affect the mental health of individuals living with HIV, and what strategies can be used to combat this stigma?

**Answer:** Stigma can lead to feelings of shame, isolation, and depression in individuals living with HIV. This can deter them from seeking care, adhering to treatment, or disclosing their status to others. To combat stigma, strategies could include community-based education programs that provide factual information about HIV and treatment, thereby reducing fear and misconceptions. For example, sharing stories of individuals living full lives with HIV can challenge stereotypes and demonstrate that people with this condition can still live long and healthy lives. Support groups also offer a safe space for individuals to share experiences and coping strategies, illustrating that a diagnosis does not define them.

**Question:** What are the potential barriers to accessing pre-exposure prophylaxis (PrEP) for HIV prevention, and how can healthcare providers address these barriers?

**Answer:** Barriers to accessing PrEP include lack of awareness, cost, stigma, and access to healthcare providers knowledgeable about PrEP. Healthcare providers can address these barriers by increasing education about PrEP among at-risk populations, advocating for cost-covering measures like insurance or patient assistance programs, and offering PrEP in a stigma-free environment. For instance, a healthcare provider might create a welcoming clinic environment with materials that feature diverse individuals discussing PrEP, signaling that it's a common and proactive health measure.

**Question:** How does cultural competency in healthcare providers improve sexual health outcomes for patients from diverse backgrounds?

**Answer:** Cultural competency involves understanding and respecting the beliefs, practices, and needs of patients from diverse backgrounds. It improves sexual health outcomes by facilitating better communication, trust, and tailored healthcare delivery. For example, a healthcare provider might offer translation services or culturally appropriate educational materials, ensuring that patients receive and understand vital sexual health information. A culturally competent provider might also be aware of specific sexual health risks or practices within certain cultures and provide relevant advice and services, such as a provider working with a patient from a culture where discussing sexual health is taboo might use more discreet and sensitive communication methods.

**Question:** What role does comprehensive sex education play in preventing adolescent pregnancies, and how should such education be structured?

**Answer:** Comprehensive sex education plays a critical role in preventing adolescent pregnancies by providing young people with accurate information about contraception, consent, and healthy relationships. Such education should be age-appropriate, medically accurate, and inclusive of all gender identities and sexual orientations. It should also empower adolescents to make informed decisions about their sexual health. For example, a comprehensive program might use interactive activities to teach about consent, provide demonstrations on the correct use of contraceptives, and encourage discussions about the emotional aspects of sexual relationships.

By providing answers focusing on person-first language and inclusive practices, we emphasize the importance of respecting and addressing individual needs, fostering a more effective and compassionate approach to sexual health education and care.

# Introducing Cohesion: A Narrative-Driven Approach to Enhancing Critical Thinking and Empathy About HIV Stigma for Healthcare Professionals

Cohesion emerges as a groundbreaking educational tool, uniquely crafted to enhance critical thinking and empathy for healthcare professionals and community advocates. At its heart, Cohesion focuses on the intricate intersection of identity and stigma, illuminated through personal narratives. This innovative approach marries accurate, relevant education with engaging, real-life scenarios, ensuring that learning is not only informative but also deeply resonant with participants' own life experiences.

## Why Cohesion Works: Engaging Hearts and Minds

The strength of Cohesion lies in its narrative-driven methodology. By weaving authentic, first-hand stories into the fabric of its training, Cohesion offers more than just theoretical knowledge; it provides a window into diverse, real-world experiences. These narratives, shared by subject matter experts who bring their own personal stories to the table, serve as powerful tools for learning. They offer participants a chance to step into another's shoes, to view the world through different lenses.

Such an immersive experience is key to fostering empathy and understanding. As participants engage with these stories, they not only learn about the complexities of identity and stigma but also develop a deeper, more nuanced appreciation of how these factors intersect with health and equity. This understanding is crucial in healthcare and advocacy, where recognizing and respecting diverse perspectives is essential for effective, compassionate care and community support.

## The Power of Reusable, Evolving Content

Another unique aspect of Cohesion is its dynamic, reusable nature. The program continually integrates fresh elements from real-life stories, ensuring that each training session remains current, relevant, and deeply engaging. This adaptability means that Cohesion is not a static learning tool but a living, evolving entity that reflects the ever-changing realities of the world we live in.

## Cultivating Critical Thinking Through Conversations

Cohesion also excels in facilitating challenging yet vital conversations. In an environment where narratives spark dialogue, participants are encouraged to think critically about complex social and health issues. This process of thoughtful exchange expands their ability to approach and tackle these challenges effectively.

## Storytelling as a Catalyst for Change

At its core, Cohesion harnesses the transformative power of storytelling to build bridges of understanding. It trains not just the mind but also the heart, equipping participants with invaluable skills to improve healthcare delivery, strengthen community bonds, and champion social justice. The unlimited potential of storytelling is harnessed to inspire positive change from within, revealing the common threads of our shared humanity.

Cohesion, therefore, is more than just a training tool—it's a pathway to deeper connection and empathy, fostering a community of informed, compassionate individuals ready to make a positive impact in their professional and personal spheres. We begin by creating our card decks.

**Objective:**

This activity is designed to help participants identify and understand key characteristics of their intended audience, fostering a deeper insight into their needs and perspectives.

**Materials Needed:**

- Five notecards per participant

**Instructions:**

1. **Initial Notecard Setup:**

   - Each participant receives five notecards.

   - On the first card, write 'PT' in the center and then flip it over.

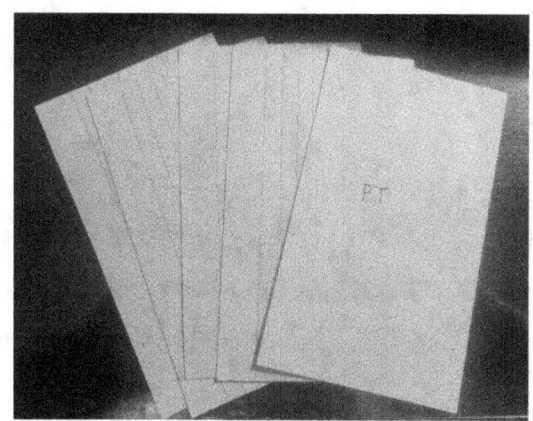

2. **Describing Audience Characteristics:**

   - On the flipped side of each notecard, at the top, write down one specific characteristic, trait, or detail about your intended audience. This could be a demographic detail, a behavioral trait, a need, or any other relevant attribute.

   - Repeat this process for all five notecards, ensuring each card highlights a different aspect of the intended audience.

3. **Completion Signal:**

   - Once you have finished detailing all the notecards, place your pen down and shift your attention towards the facilitator as a signal of completion. See my deck as an example.

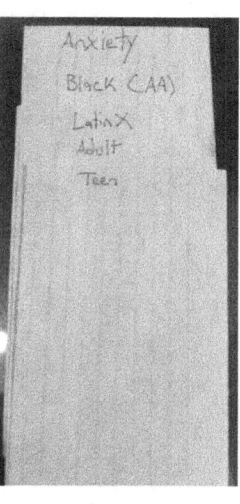

4. **Exchanging Decks:**

   - Pass your entire deck of PT notecards to another participant randomly.

   - Receive a PT deck from another participant.

5. **Adding Additional Perspectives:**

   - On the deck you received, read the characteristic or detail at the top of each card.

   - Then, at the bottom of each card, add another trait or detail about the intended audience as you perceive it. Do not use the same descriptions that are on these 5 cards. What you choose should be entirely new descriptions for this deck. See the deck below as an example.

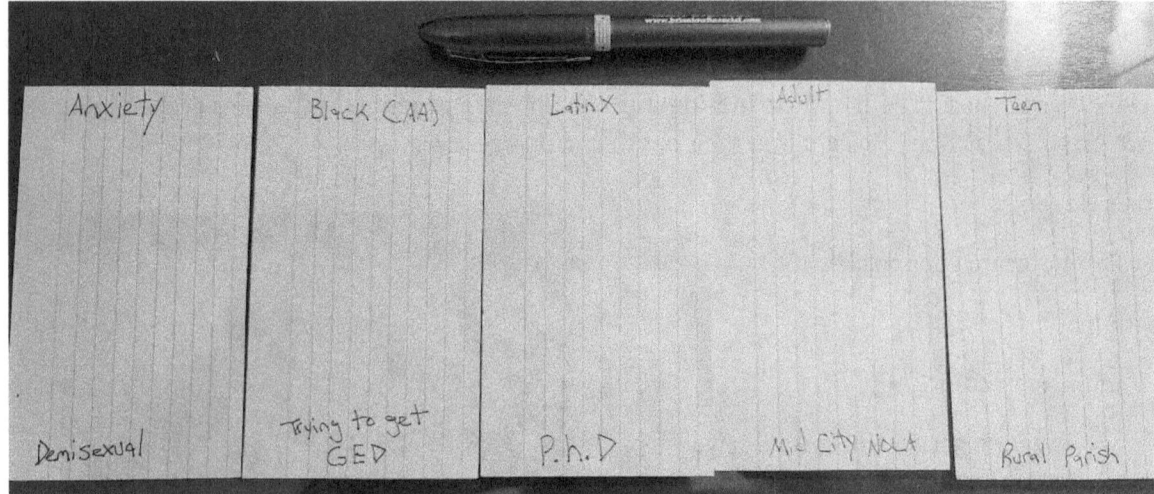

- This step enriches the deck with diverse perspectives on the same audience.

6. **Finalizing the Deck:**

   - After adding your contributions to the notecards, write 'PT' on the back of each card.

   - Once completed, place your pen down and direct your attention back to the facilitator.

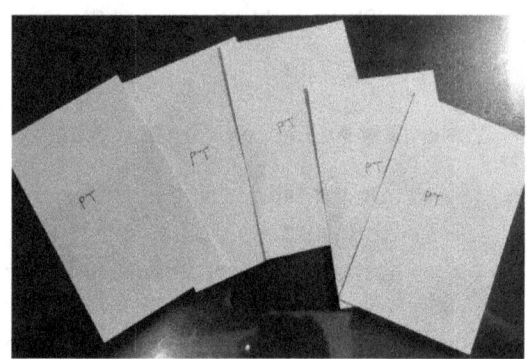

**Outcome:**

This activity equips participants with the skills to collaboratively create a detailed profile of their target audience, thereby deepening their understanding and enhancing their ability to effectively meet the audience's needs. A key objective is to foster comfort and fluency in discussing symptoms and medical conditions. By normalizing these conversations, participants can practice and refine their communication skills, essential for creating a stigma-free environment. This approach is crucial in healthcare settings, as it encourages clients to seek timely treatment by offering them a safe space to discuss their health concerns openly and without fear of judgment.

Audience Characteristics Example Table 1 - Two Decks of Examples

| Audience Category | Characteristic/Trait/Detail | Description/Example |
| --- | --- | --- |
| Demographic Details | Age | Specific age group (e.g., Teens, Adults over 50) |
| | Gender | Gender identity (e.g., Male, Female, Non-Binary) |

| Audience Category | Characteristic/Trait/Detail | Description/Example |
|---|---|---|
| | Location | Geographic location (e.g., Urban, Rural, Specific region) |
| | Education Level | Highest level of education attained (e.g., High School, College) |
| | Socioeconomic Status | Income level, occupation, social class (e.g., Low-income, Middle-class) |
| Behavioral Traits | Lifestyle | Type of lifestyle (e.g., Active, Sedentary, Nomadic) |
| | Interests/Hobbies | Specific interests or hobbies (e.g., Sports, Arts, Technology) |
| | Consumer Habits | Shopping and consumption patterns (e.g., Online shopper, Budget-conscious) |
| | Communication Preferences | Preferred modes of communication (e.g., Email, Social Media, In-person) |
| Needs | Health Needs | Specific health-related needs (e.g., Chronic illness management, Mental health support) |
| | Educational Needs | Learning requirements (e.g., Continued education, Literacy programs) |
| | Emotional Support | Types of emotional support needed (e.g., Counseling, Peer support groups) |
| | Accessibility Requirements | Needs for physical or digital accessibility (e.g., Wheelchair access, Screen reader-friendly content) |
| Other Attributes | Cultural Background | Cultural or ethnic background (e.g., Hispanic, Asian-American) |
| | Language Preferences | Preferred language(s) for communication (e.g., English, Spanish, ASL) |
| | Technology Usage | Level of comfort and frequency of technology use (e.g., Tech-savvy, Limited tech use) |

This table format helps in structuring a detailed and organized profile of an intended audience, capturing various aspects that are crucial for understanding their characteristics and needs. This can be particularly useful in tailoring communication strategies, services, or products to meet the specific requirements of different audience groups.

Below is a table that outlines how specific characteristics and traits of certain audiences are often expressed. This table can provide insights into understanding and identifying these characteristics in real-world contexts:

Audience Characteristics Example Table 2 - Two Decks of Examples

| Audience Category | Characteristic/Trait/Detail | How Often Expressed/Manifested |
|---|---|---|
| Demographic Details | Age | Preferences in entertainment, clothing, technology use; specific health concerns or priorities. |
| | Gender | Choice of products or services, participation in certain activities, communication style. |
| | Location | Localized cultural references, responses to climate or regional events, local dialects or slang. |
| | Education Level | Types of literature or media consumed, engagement in intellectual or academic discussions, vocabulary use. |
| | Socioeconomic Status | Shopping habits, leisure activities, financial priorities or constraints. |
| Behavioral Traits | Lifestyle | Social media content, leisure activities, types of events attended, daily routines. |
| | Interests/Hobbies | Membership in related clubs or groups, types of books or magazines read, related social media groups or content. |
| | Consumer Habits | Brand loyalty, shopping frequency, responses to marketing or advertising. |
| | Communication Preferences | Preferred channels for receiving information, responsiveness to different media formats, level of formality in communication. |
| Needs | Health Needs | Seeking information related to specific health conditions, usage of certain healthcare services, involvement in related support groups. |
| | Educational Needs | Participation in educational programs or workshops, type of content shared or interacted with online. |

| Audience Category | Characteristic/Trait/Detail | How Often Expressed/Manifested |
|---|---|---|
| | Emotional Support | Engagement with self-help or motivational content, participation in counseling or therapy, involvement in peer support groups. |
| | Accessibility Requirements | Use of assistive technologies, feedback on accessibility features, specific requests for accommodations. |
| Other Attributes | Cultural Background | Preferences in food, entertainment, participation in cultural events, language usage. |
| | Language Preferences | Choice of media, responsiveness to multilingual content, engagement in community/language-specific groups. |
| | Technology Usage | Frequency and type of device usage, engagement with tech-related content, proficiency in using digital platforms. |

This table helps in understanding how various audience characteristics are typically expressed, which is crucial for identifying and effectively engaging with different groups. It can guide the development of tailored communication strategies, services, or products to better meet the specific needs and preferences of diverse audiences.

Facilitated Debrief: Discussing PT Card Choices and Addressing Biases

**Introduction:**

As we wrap up the activity with the Population and Target Audience (PT) cards, let's take this opportunity for a crucial debrief. I encourage everyone to engage openly and thoughtfully in this discussion.

**Understanding Our Choices:**

☐ **Share Your Choices:**

   o Let's go around the room, and I'd like each of you to share one trait or descriptor you wrote on your PT cards. Explain why you chose it. What story or perspective were you aiming to capture?

☐ **Reflecting on Our Decisions:**

   o As you listen to each other, think about the reasons behind these choices. Were they based on personal experiences, societal perceptions, or something else?

**Addressing Internal Biases:**

- ❑ **Recognizing Bias:**

  - o It's natural to have preconceived notions or biases. If you felt any internal resistance or bias while writing down certain traits, let's talk about that. This is a safe space for honest reflection.

- ❑ **Impact of Bias on Care:**

  - o Discuss how these biases, if unchecked, could influence our interactions with clients. How might they affect the care we provide?

## Exploring the Stories Behind the Descriptors:

- ❑ **Beyond the Descriptors:**

  - o Remember, descriptors are just one part of a person's story. If you're comfortable, share a personal descriptor about yourself, like I did with being tired or having episodic headaches. How does this descriptor fit into your larger story?

- ❑ **Normalizing Diversity in Healthcare Needs:**

  - o How can we use this understanding to better empathize with and support our clients? How do we ensure we're seeing the whole person and not just a set of symptoms or traits?

## Encouraging Holistic Viewpoints:

- ■ **Everyone Has a Story:**

  - o Reflect on the idea that everyone, including ourselves, has aspects that require care and assistance. How does this influence our approach to healthcare?

- ■ **No One is an Island:**

  - o Discuss the importance of support and community in healthcare. How can we foster an environment where clients feel understood and not isolated because of their conditions or traits?

## Concluding Thoughts:

Today's discussion serves as a pivotal instrument for our continuous professional growth. The perspectives and insights exchanged here are invaluable in bolstering our empathy, deepening our understanding, and refining our effectiveness as healthcare professionals. Such dialogues are essential for our evolution, both as individuals and as a united team, dedicated to delivering care that is not only comprehensive but infused with compassion and understanding. Let's carry forward the lessons learned today, allowing them to shape and enhance our approach to healthcare, ensuring we always see and treat our clients as whole, multifaceted individuals.

## Creating Your Medical Condition (MC) Deck

**Objective:** This component of the workshop involves creating a personalized Medical Condition (MC) Deck to enhance participants' awareness of various medical conditions and their relevance to specific populations.

**Instructions:**

1.  **Introduction to MC Deck:**

    - Introduce the Medical Condition (MC) Deck as a tool for understanding a range of medical conditions that may affect the populations you serve, such as HIV, STIs, TB, HCV, and others.

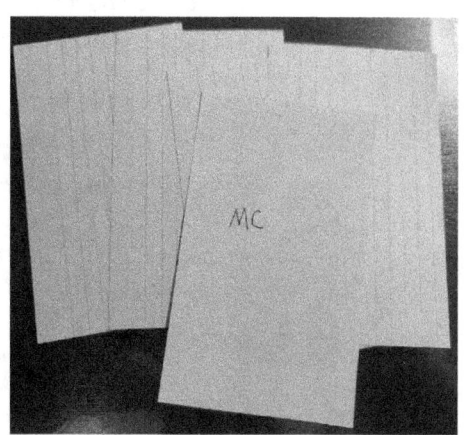

2.  **Selection of Conditions:**

    - Each participant receives five notecards.

    - On the first card, write 'MC' in the center and then flip it over.

    - Each participant will select 5 medical conditions, which they believe are significant to their target audience.

    - Label the top of each notecard with one condition or a combination of conditions that you deem relevant. For example, the first card might read 'HIV', the second 'HIV, Herpes, HCV', and the third 'HIV, HCV'. Check out my deck as an example.

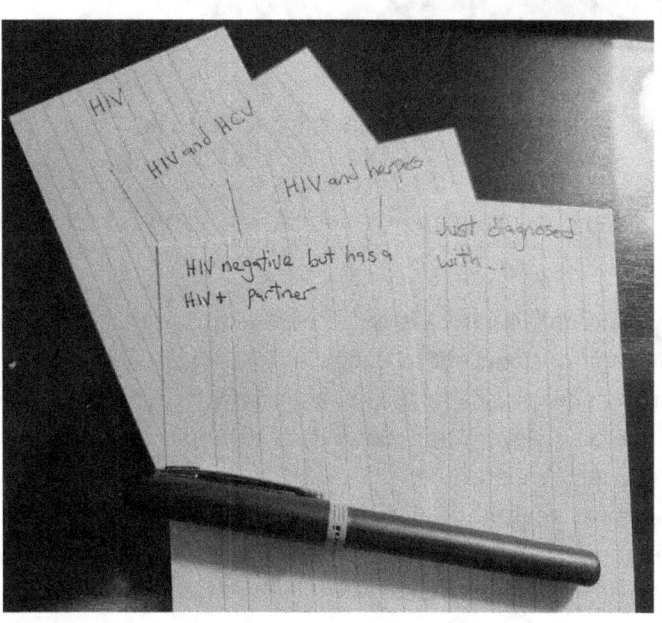

3.  **Completion and Attention Signal:**

    - After labeling all your notecards, set your pen down as a signal that you have completed this step and are ready to proceed.

- Turn your focus to the facilitator for further instructions.

4. **Exchange and Speculation:**

   - Pass your set of MC notecards to another participant in a random manner.

   - Upon receiving a set of MC notecards from another participant, review the conditions listed and speculate on additional medical conditions that could be pertinent to the target population noted. Write these on the bottom of each card.

   - Do not use the same descriptions that are on these 5 cards. What you choose should be entirely new descriptions for this deck. See the deck below as an example.

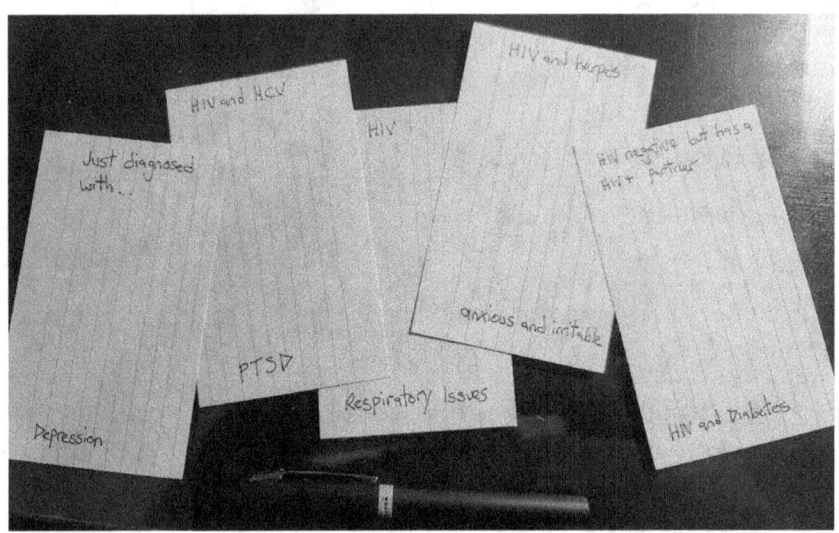

5. **Finalization:**

   - Once completed, flip each notecard over and mark the back with 'MC' to indicate the deck's theme.

   - Set your pen down again and direct your attention to the facilitator to indicate you are ready to move on.

**Outcome:** Participating in the Medical Condition (MC) Deck exercise enables participants to develop a deep understanding of various medical conditions relevant to their clientele. The goal is to enhance participants' abilities to empathize with and effectively address the health needs of those they serve. A key objective is to become comfortable discussing symptoms and details of medical conditions in everyday conversations. This exercise facilitates the practice of these skills, helping participants normalize discussions around health topics. As healthcare professionals, it's vital to communicate these matters in a relaxed and comfortable manner, thereby creating a welcoming space for clients to openly discuss their health issues. This approach is crucial in addressing the stigma that often leads people to delay seeking treatment.

Below is a table that details specific characteristics and traits associated with different health conditions, both individually and in combination. This table can be used to understand the complex nature of these conditions and their impact on individuals:

Medical Condition Table 1 - Two Decks of Examples

| Condition(s) | Specific Characteristics | Traits/Impact on Individuals |
|---|---|---|
| HIV | Virus affecting the immune system. | Chronic management, possible social stigma, regular medical care, and antiretroviral therapy. |
| HIV, Herpes | Combination of HIV and Herpes (a common viral infection). | In addition to HIV traits, periodic herpes outbreaks, requiring antiviral treatment. |
| HIV, HCV (Hepatitis C) | Co-infection with HIV and Hepatitis C. | Increased liver-related health issues, complex treatment regimen, heightened stigma. |
| Herpes | Virus causing sores on mouth or genitals. | Recurrent outbreaks, stigma associated with sexual transmission, manageable with medication. |
| HCV | Viral infection causing liver inflammation, potentially chronic. | Long-term health implications, possible liver damage, treatable with antiviral drugs. |
| HIV, TB (Tuberculosis) | HIV co-infected with Tuberculosis. | Complicated treatment due to weakened immune system, increased risk of TB activation. |
| Diabetes | Chronic condition affecting blood sugar regulation. | Lifestyle modifications, regular monitoring, potential for long-term complications. |
| HIV, Diabetes | HIV combined with Diabetes. | Managing two chronic conditions, interactions between treatments, comprehensive care required. |
| Asthma | Chronic respiratory condition causing breathing difficulty. | Trigger management, use of inhalers, impact on daily activities and physical exertion. |
| HIV, Asthma | HIV co-existing with Asthma. | Managing respiratory challenges along with HIV, potential medication interactions. |
| HCV, Diabetes | Hepatitis C co-existing with Diabetes. | Liver health monitoring, blood sugar management, potential for compounded complications. |

| Condition(s) | Specific Characteristics | Traits/Impact on Individuals |
|---|---|---|
| Herpes, TB | Co-occurrence of Herpes and Tuberculosis. | Managing recurrent herpes outbreaks and TB treatment, potential for weakened immune response. |

This table is intended to provide a detailed overview of various health conditions, either individually or in combination, focusing on their specific characteristics and the traits or impacts they may have on individuals. Understanding these nuances is crucial for healthcare professionals and others working with affected populations to provide appropriate care and support.

Below is a detailed table focusing on how specific characteristics and traits of various health conditions, both individually and in combination, are often expressed:

Medical Condition Table 2 - Two Decks of Examples

| Condition(s) | Characteristic/Trait | How Often Expressed/Manifested |
|---|---|---|
| HIV | Immune System Compromise | Frequent illnesses, slow recovery, specific opportunistic infections like thrush or pneumonia. |
| | Medication Regimen | Daily antiretroviral therapy, regular medical appointments, strict adherence to medication schedules. |
| HIV, Herpes | Recurrent Outbreaks | Periodic sores or blisters, usually triggered by stress or immune system changes, alongside HIV symptoms. |
| | Dual Medication Management | Balancing antiretroviral therapy with antiviral treatment for herpes, managing potential drug interactions. |
| HIV, HCV | Liver Health Concerns | Elevated liver enzymes, potential jaundice, alongside symptoms of HIV. |
| | Complex Treatment | Combining HIV treatment with HCV therapy, monitoring for liver toxicity. |
| Herpes | Visible Sores | Periodic outbreaks of sores, typically on mouth or genitals, triggered by various factors. |
| | Stigma | Social stigma related to sexual transmission, impacting mental and emotional health. |
| HCV | Liver Function Impairment | Fatigue, jaundice, abdominal pain, often unnoticed until significant liver damage occurs. |

| Condition(s) | Characteristic/Trait | How Often Expressed/Manifested |
| --- | --- | --- |
| HIV, TB | Asymptomatic Nature | Long periods without symptoms, often leading to delayed diagnosis and treatment. |
| | Respiratory Issues | Coughing, chest pain, breathing difficulties, alongside symptoms of HIV. |
| | Co-management of Conditions | Combining TB treatment with HIV therapy, monitoring for interactions and side effects. |
| Diabetes | Blood Sugar Fluctuations | Frequent urination, thirst, fatigue, blurred vision, risk of hypoglycemia or hyperglycemia. |
| | Lifestyle Adjustments | Dietary changes, regular exercise, blood sugar monitoring, possibly insulin therapy. |
| HIV, Diabetes | Multi-faceted Health Management | Managing blood sugar alongside HIV treatment, increased monitoring for complications. |
| | Medication Adherence and Interactions | Balancing HIV medication with diabetes treatment, vigilant about interactions and side effects. |
| Asthma | Breathing Difficulties | Shortness of breath, wheezing, coughing, particularly during physical activity or allergen exposure. |
| | Trigger Management | Avoidance of allergens, use of inhalers, need for emergency medication in severe cases. |
| HIV, Asthma | Compound Respiratory Challenges | Managing asthma symptoms alongside potential respiratory infections due to HIV. |
| | Coordinated Care Requirements | Balancing asthma management with HIV treatment, monitoring lung health closely. |
| HCV, Diabetes | Liver and Blood Sugar Management | Monitoring and managing liver health in conjunction with blood sugar levels, lifestyle adjustments. |
| | Integrated Healthcare Approach | Coordinated care for both conditions, regular health check-ups, and holistic treatment strategies. |
| Herpes, TB | Immune System Strain | Managing both respiratory symptoms of TB and periodic herpes outbreaks, increased immune challenges. |
| | Comprehensive Treatment Approach | Coordinating treatment for both conditions, monitoring for side effects and interactions. |

This table illustrates how different health conditions and their combinations are expressed through various symptoms, lifestyle impacts, and treatment requirements. Understanding these expressions is crucial for healthcare providers and caregivers in delivering appropriate care and support to individuals with these conditions.

Facilitated Debrief: Exploring Choices and Challenging Biases in the MC Cards Exercise

**Introduction:**

"Thank you all for participating in the Medical Condition (MC) Deck exercise. Now, let's take some time to reflect and discuss our choices and the thoughts that guided them. This debrief is a safe space for open conversation about the traits and conditions we chose to include on our cards, and more importantly, why we chose them.

**Encouraging Sharing of Choices:**

- **Sharing Individual Selections:**
    - "Let's start by sharing what each of us wrote on our MC cards. Don't hesitate to explain why you chose those specific conditions or traits."
    - "Remember, there's no right or wrong here. This is about understanding our thought processes and learning from each other."

- **Discussing Underlying Reasons:**
    - "As we share, let's delve into the reasons behind our choices. Were they based on personal experiences, common conditions, or perhaps conditions we find challenging to address?"

- **Addressing Awkwardness and Discomfort:**
    - "If you felt awkward writing down certain traits, let's talk about that. It's important to explore any discomfort we might feel, as it can be an indicator of underlying biases or gaps in our understanding."

**Exploring Internal Biases:**

- **Recognizing and Discussing Biases:**
    - "If any of us noticed an internal bias while making these cards, now is the time to bring it to light. It's crucial we address these biases here, rather than in front of our clients."
    - "Discussing our biases openly can help us understand and overcome them, leading to more compassionate and effective care."

- **Sharing Concerns and Anxieties:**

o "Were there any worries or concerns that came up during this exercise? It's natural to feel uncertain, especially when dealing with complex medical conditions."

**Examples of Internal Bias and Addressing Them in a Group Setting:**

✂ **Bias Based on Appearance or Lifestyle Choices:**

    o **Example:** A healthcare professional might realize they have preconceived notions about individuals with tattoos or piercings, assuming they are less responsible or more likely to engage in risky behaviors.

    o **Addressing in Group:** Encourage open discussion about why such stereotypes exist and how they can be harmful. Emphasize the importance of treating each client as an individual, not as a stereotype.

✂ **Bias Related to Mental Health:**

    o **Example:** A participant might notice they hold a bias that people with mental health issues, such as depression, are always visibly sad or unable to function effectively.

    o **Addressing in Group:** Discuss the spectrum of mental health and the varied ways it can manifest. Stress the need for healthcare professionals to approach mental health with the same seriousness and lack of judgment as physical health.

✂ **Socioeconomic Bias:**

    o **Example:** An implicit assumption that individuals from lower socioeconomic backgrounds might be less knowledgeable about health issues or less compliant with treatment plans.

    o **Addressing in Group:** Explore how socioeconomic factors influence access to healthcare and education. Encourage empathy and understanding that compliance often relates to resources and access, not just personal choice.

✂ **Cultural or Racial Bias:**

    o **Example:** A team member might recognize an unconscious bias in assuming certain cultural or racial groups have specific health behaviors or attitudes towards health.

    o **Addressing in Group:** Facilitate a conversation about cultural competency and the dangers of generalizing based on race or culture. Highlight the importance of individualized care that respects and incorporates each person's cultural background.

✂ **Age-Related Bias:**

    o **Example:** Believing younger clients are less likely to take their health seriously or that older clients are resistant to change or new technologies.

- **Addressing in Group:** Address age stereotypes and discuss the individual variability within age groups. Emphasize the need to approach clients of all ages with openness and without preconceived notions.

**Bias Towards Individuals with Substance Use History:**

- **Example:** An internal bias that individuals with a history of substance use are less reliable or trustworthy.
- **Addressing in Group:** Openly discuss the nature of addiction as a health issue and the stigma that often surrounds it. Promote understanding and compassion in treatment approaches.

In addressing these biases, the key is to create an environment where group members feel safe to express and examine their biases without judgment. This fosters a culture of learning and growth, encouraging healthcare professionals to provide more equitable and sensitive care.

**Reflecting on Descriptors and Human Complexity:**

1. **Understanding Descriptors as Part of a Larger Story:**
    - "Consider my own descriptors – tired, knees crackling, episodic headaches. These traits could align with various conditions, or none at all. They're pieces of a larger story, not definitive labels."
    - "It's crucial to remember that these descriptors are not the entirety of a person's story. Each individual is more than their condition or traits."
2. **Emphasizing Holistic Care:**
    - "Let's remind ourselves that we all have aspects of ourselves that require care, assistance, and encouragement. Recognizing this helps us provide more holistic and empathetic care."
3. **No One is an Island:**
    - "Acknowledging that no one is an island reinforces the need for community, support, and understanding in healthcare. It's essential in our approach to client care."

**Conclusion:**

"Today's discussion marks a crucial step in enhancing our approach to healthcare. It has underscored the importance of empathy, a deep understanding of our clients' experiences, and a keen awareness of our own perceptions and biases. As we move forward, let's actively integrate these insights into our daily practice, constantly aiming to offer the highest standard of care to all our clients. This commitment to self-awareness and empathetic engagement is key to delivering truly comprehensive and compassionate healthcare services."

**Overview:** The Age and Diagnostic Setting (ADS) Deck is a dynamic and educational tool crafted to illustrate the wide range of ages and various settings where individuals might encounter medical diagnoses. This tool aims to enhance understanding of how different environments and life stages impact the diagnosis experience and healthcare needs.

**Instructions for ADS Activity:**

1. **Setup:**

   - Each participant receives a set of five cards specifically for this activity.

   - On the first card, write 'ADS' in the center and then flip it over.

2. **Card Preparation:**

   - Your primary objective in this activity is to depict not only the age but also the stage of maturity at which an individual might receive a medical diagnosis, paired with the appropriate diagnostic setting. If your existing decks already include specific ages or age ranges, you can further enhance this by focusing on the key developmental stages the individual is experiencing at the time of diagnosis. For instance, the first age card might indicate a specific age, such as '30 years old, at a specialist clinic', signifying an adult in their prime possibly facing a chronic condition diagnosis.

     Each card is designed to provide an in-depth exploration of the individual's developmental stage, such as 'early adulthood, navigating independence and career'. This approach offers a more comprehensive view of the individual's life circumstances and the challenges they face at the time of their diagnosis, moving beyond mere chronological age. It illuminates the unique challenges and needs they may encounter during their medical journey, and draws attention to competing life priorities that may impact their response to and management of their diagnosis. This deeper understanding is invaluable for healthcare professionals, fostering empathy and aiding them in guiding their clients toward making informed treatment decisions.

   - On the top of each card, detail an age, followed by a specific diagnostic setting. For example, Card 1 could read '25, Emergency Room', illustrating a young adult possibly facing an acute medical issue. In contrast, Card 2 might read '5, Family Doctor's Office', depicting a young child at a routine check-up or facing a common childhood illness. This nuanced approach ensures a holistic view of the patient's situation, emphasizing the interplay between their life stage, health condition, and the healthcare environment. If you get stuck just imagine why they may be receiving medical care at that moment.

   - See the tables at the end of this section for assistance with descriptions and individual developmental stages.

   **Labeling the Deck:**

   - After annotating the top of all five cards, flip the entire deck over.

- Write 'ADS' on the back of the first card to identify the deck's theme.

3. **Exchange and Collaboration:**

   - Once you have completed your part, exchange your deck with another participant chosen at random.

   - The next person will add their suggested age and setting at the bottom of each card. Do not use the same descriptions that are on these 5 cards. What you choose should be entirely new descriptions for this deck.

   - If it's difficult to think of the setting, simply imagine where you, your child, or your family members would have contact with medical care and they might run routine testing.

4. **Finalizing the Cards:**

   - After the additional information is added, flip the cards back over.

   - Write 'ADS' on the back of the remaining cards to complete the deck.

**Purpose of the Activity:** This exercise aims to broaden participants' understanding of the variety in age and setting related to medical diagnoses. It fosters empathy and enhances awareness of the varied experiences patients go through during their diagnostic journeys. Through this collaborative activity, participants gain a deeper insight into the multifaceted nature of patient experiences in healthcare settings.

We encourage you to explore the tables below that go along with this section.

Below is a detailed table showcasing specific characteristics and traits associated with various ages and diagnostic settings for health conditions:

Age and Diagnostic Setting Table 1 - Two Decks of Examples

| Card Number | Age and Setting | Characteristic/Trait of Diagnosis | Description/Context |
|---|---|---|---|
| 1 | 25, Emergency Room | Acute Condition Detection | Likely scenarios include accidents, acute illness symptoms, or sudden health complications. |
| 2 | 5, Family Doctor's Office | Early Childhood Illness or Condition | Common for routine check-ups, vaccinations, or identifying developmental health issues. |
| 3 | 30, Specialist Clinic | Chronic Condition Diagnosis | Age where certain chronic conditions like diabetes or thyroid issues might first be noticed. |

| Card Number | Age and Setting | Characteristic/Trait of Diagnosis | Description/Context |
|---|---|---|---|
| 4 | 60, Hospital | Late-Onset Condition Diagnosis | Common for detecting conditions like heart disease, cancer, or late-onset diabetes. |
| 5 | 18, University Health Center | Young Adult Health Concerns | Mental health issues, sexual health concerns, or lifestyle-related conditions are typical. |
| 6 | 45, Community Health Center | Midlife Health Screenings | Routine screenings for conditions prevalent in middle age, like hypertension or cholesterol. |
| 7 | 70, Geriatric Clinic | Geriatric-Specific Conditions | Age-related conditions like Alzheimer's, osteoporosis, or age-related macular degeneration. |
| 8 | 16, Pediatrician | Adolescent Health Issues | Issues like hormonal changes, growth concerns, or adolescent mental health. |
| 9 | 35, Obstetrics/Gynecology Clinic | Reproductive Health Concerns | Common for pregnancy-related check-ups or reproductive health issues. |
| 10 | 50, Oncology Center | Cancer Screening and Diagnosis | Age where the risk for certain types of cancer increases, leading to more frequent screenings. |

This table provides a framework for understanding how age and diagnostic setting play a crucial role in the type of health conditions typically diagnosed and the context in which these diagnoses occur. It can be used as a guide for healthcare professionals, educators, and individuals to better understand the healthcare needs and concerns at different life stages and in various healthcare settings.

Below is a detailed table focusing on how specific characteristics and traits related to age and diagnostic setting are often expressed:

Age and Diagnostic Setting Table 2 – Two Decks of Example Expressions

| Card Number | Age and Setting | How Characteristics/Traits are Expressed |
|---|---|---|
| 1 | 25, Emergency Room | Sudden, acute symptoms requiring immediate attention; often results from accidents, severe infections, or acute health crises. |
| 2 | 5, Family Doctor's Office | Common childhood illnesses or developmental issues identified during routine check-ups or vaccinations. |
| 3 | 30, Specialist Clinic | Identification of chronic conditions through specialized tests, often following referral due to persistent symptoms. |
| 4 | 60, Hospital | Diagnosis of late-onset conditions often in response to emergency symptoms or during routine screenings for age-related diseases. |
| 5 | 18, University Health Center | Health concerns typical of young adulthood, such as mental health issues or lifestyle-related conditions, often brought up during campus life. |
| 6 | 45, Community Health Center | Midlife health screenings for conditions like hypertension, often during regular health check-ups or as a part of preventive health care. |
| 7 | 70, Geriatric Clinic | Diagnosis of geriatric conditions, typically during routine visits, focusing on age-related diseases and managing multiple health issues. |
| 8 | 16, Pediatrician | Adolescent-specific health issues, often addressed during regular check-ups or as a result of growth and hormonal changes. |
| 9 | 35, Obstetrics/Gynecology Clinic | Issues related to reproductive health, often expressed during routine exams or as a result of pregnancy and related health concerns. |
| 10 | 50, Oncology Center | Concerns related to cancer, often expressed during specialized screenings or in response to specific symptoms indicative of cancer. |

This table illustrates how the combination of age and diagnostic setting influences the expression of health concerns and the manner in which they are addressed. It provides a framework for understanding the typical health scenarios encountered in different settings and at various stages of life, aiding in anticipation and preparation for these situations.

Table 3 provides an in-depth exploration of individual developmental stages, ages, and corresponding diagnostic settings as they might appear in the Age and Diagnostic Setting (ADS) deck.

Age and Diagnostic Setting Table 3 – Individual Developmental Stages Examples

| Developmental Stage | Age | Diagnostic Setting | In-depth Exploration |
|---|---|---|---|
| Early Childhood | 3 | Pediatrician's Office | Focus on developmental milestones, common childhood illnesses, immunizations, and early detection of any developmental disorders. |
| Late Childhood | 10 | School Health Clinic | Addressing school-related health issues, mental wellness, social development, and early signs of learning disabilities or behavioral concerns. |
| Adolescence | 16 | Adolescent Health Center | Navigating puberty, sexual health education, mental health screenings, and addressing risk-taking behaviors typical in adolescence. |
| Early Adulthood | 25 | Emergency Room | Possible acute medical issues or injuries, mental health crises, or the onset of chronic conditions like hypertension or Type 2 diabetes. |
| Midlife | 45 | General Practitioner's Office | Routine screenings for chronic diseases, managing stress related to career or family, and addressing the onset of menopause or andropause. |
| Early Senior Years | 65 | Specialty Clinic (e.g., Cardiology) | Focusing on age-related conditions such as heart disease, diabetes management, and screenings for cancers. |
| Advanced Age | 80 | Geriatric Clinic | Addressing complex health needs, multi-morbidity management, dementia or Alzheimer's screenings, and discussions about long-term care planning. |
| Palliative Stage | Any Age | Hospice or Palliative Care | Providing comfort care, pain management, and emotional support for terminal illnesses, tailored to the individual's and family's needs. |

This table encapsulates how the ADS deck can represent the varying developmental stages, corresponding ages, and appropriate diagnostic settings. Each entry provides insights into the specific health concerns, screenings, and typical medical interactions relevant to that stage of life. This approach aims to create a holistic understanding of an individual's health journey across different stages of life, ensuring healthcare professionals can provide age and stage-appropriate care and support.

**Introduction:**

As we wrap up our session involving the Age and Diagnostic Setting (ADS) cards, I invite all of us to participate in a reflective debriefing. This is an opportunity for open and honest dialogue in a supportive and safe environment. Your active participation is not only encouraged but essential to the richness of our discussion. Let's take this time to share insights, reflect on our learning, and understand the diverse perspectives that have emerged from this exercise.

**Discussion of Choices:**

1. **Sharing Your ADS Card Choices:**

    - Let's start by sharing the age and diagnostic setting you chose for your ADS cards. What influenced your decision? Was it personal experience, societal observations, or something else?

2. **Understanding the Context:**

    - Reflect on the broader context of the age and setting you selected. How do these factors influence the patient experience and the approach to care?

**Addressing Internal Biases:**

1. **Recognizing and Discussing Biases:**

    - If you noticed any internal biases or discomfort while selecting certain ages or settings, let's discuss these feelings. Why do you think these biases exist, and how can we address them?

2. **Impact on Patient Care:**

    - Consider how these biases, if unacknowledged, might affect our interactions with patients. How can we ensure our biases do not influence the quality of care provided?

**Exploring Descriptors and Stories:**

1. **Beyond the Descriptors:**

    - Think about the descriptors we use to categorize patients. Share a personal descriptor, much like I shared about being tired or having headaches. How does this descriptor fit into your story?

2. **Normalizing Health Discussions:**

    - How can we use our understanding of descriptors to empathize with our patients? Discuss how we can communicate that everyone has unique health needs and deserves care and support.

**Fostering a Holistic Viewpoint:**

1. **Recognizing Every Story:**

- Reflect on the idea that everyone has a unique health journey. How does this shape our approach to healthcare?

2. **The Importance of Support:**

    - Discuss the role of support in healthcare. How can we create an environment where patients feel understood and not isolated due to their conditions or age?

**Conclusion:**

Let's embrace this discussion as a pivotal moment for personal and professional development. The perspectives and understanding we've cultivated today are crucial in deepening our empathy and sharpening our skills as healthcare providers. It's important to remember that our role extends beyond mere treatment; it encompasses a comprehensive understanding and support of our patients' overall well-being. In the realm of healthcare, acknowledging the entire range of human experiences is fundamental to delivering truly compassionate and holistic care. No individual exists in isolation, and our recognition of this interconnectedness is vital in fostering a nurturing and empathetic healthcare environment.

## Creating Your Social Support Network (SSN) Deck

**Objective:** The purpose of this exercise is to intricately explore and understand the diverse range of social support systems that individuals may access following a medical diagnosis. It highlights the varying degrees of support these networks can provide, from emotional and practical assistance to professional healthcare support. This activity aims to deepen participants' insights into how different types of social support play a crucial role in an individual's journey through healthcare and recovery. By recognizing and categorizing these support systems, participants can better appreciate their significance and learn to integrate this understanding into their professional practice.

**Materials Needed:**

- Notecards (5 per participant).

**Instructions:**

1. **Initial Setup:**

2. Provide each participant with five notecards. Instruct them to turn over one of these notecards and write "SSN" (Social Support Network) on the back. Then, have them flip the card back to its front side, preparing it for the next step of the activity.

**Identifying Support Networks:**

- Participants are to write down on the top of each notecard a type of social support that exists in either their own lives or in the life of a hypothetical patient or client. This support should be one that can aid in managing a medical diagnosis and the accompanying stigma. Key figures in this social support network may also be involved in the delicate process of status disclosure. Potential sources of support to consider include family members, friends, healthcare providers, support groups, and various other resources. Each notecard should represent a different facet of this support system, capturing the diversity and complexity of the networks that assist individuals in navigating their healthcare journeys.

3. **Rating Support Level:**

   - Rate the level of support offered by each resource, writing this at the bottom of the same notecard. Use a scale of 1 to 5, where 1 indicates minimal support and 5 indicates very strong support. Seek to include a range that is an honest assessment.

4. **Preparing for Exchange:**

   - Once all notecards are completed, participants should place their pens down, signaling readiness for the next phase.

5. **First Round of Sharing Cards:**

   - Pass your set of notecards randomly to another participant.

6. **Adding Perspectives:**

   - On receiving another participant's notecards, read their identified support type. Add an additional type of support at the bottom of each card. Then, rate the effectiveness of this new support (written at the bottom) at the top of the card, using the 1 to 5 scale.

   - Seek to choose should be entirely new support types for this deck.

7. **Finalizing the Card:**

   - After adding your contributions and ratings, flip each card over and label the back with "SSN" to signify the deck's theme.

8. **Concluding the Activity:**

   - Once finished, place your pen down and look towards the facilitator as a signal of completion.

9. **Second Round of Sharing Cards:**

   - Again, pass your notecards randomly to a different participant if the group intends to engage in the storytelling exercise.

**Introduction to Group Discussion:**

After finishing the two rounds of labeling the Social Support Network (SSN) cards, let's gather for an insightful group discussion. This is a chance to collectively reflect on our findings and share perspectives.

   o **Diversity in Social Support:**

- Reflect on the wide range of social supports we identified. What types of support stood out to you, and why?

- Consider the varying levels of effectiveness you assigned. How did you determine these ratings, and what factors influenced your decisions?

  o **Role of Support Networks in Stigma and Recovery:**

- Discuss how a strong support network can be crucial in overcoming stigma associated with health conditions.

- Share thoughts on how different types of support can contribute uniquely to an individual's recovery process.

  o **The Experience of Disclosure:**

- Imagine disclosing a health condition to each type of social support you listed. Reflect on what it would feel like, considering the effectiveness rating you provided.

- How might the level of support impact one's willingness to disclose or discuss their health concerns?

- Share any personal experiences or observations that might shed light on the disclosure process.


**Conclusion:**

- Summarize the key insights gained from this discussion.

- Emphasize the importance of understanding and fostering diverse forms of social support in healthcare and recovery.

**Outcome:** The purpose of this exercise is to broaden participants' understanding of the diverse age groups and settings in which medical diagnoses occur. It aims to nurture empathy and deepen recognition of the varied experiences that patients encounter during their diagnostic and treatment journey. Through this collaborative exercise, participants will develop a nuanced understanding of the intricate stories inherent in different healthcare environments.

This activity focuses on more than just identifying social support figures; it delves into the complexities of disclosing and communicating health issues with key people in a patient's life. It acknowledges that not everyone possesses the same resources or feels safe to openly communicate their health status. In regions with mandatory disclosure laws, understanding how to effectively communicate a diagnosis becomes even more crucial, as it can profoundly impact a client's mental and emotional well-being.

The overarching goal is to enhance the participants' ability to empathize with and adeptly address the needs of a wide array of populations. This exercise is designed to facilitate comfort in discussing symptoms and medical conditions as a routine aspect of conversations. By providing a practice ground for these vital communication skills, it aims to normalize discussions around health and wellness.

For healthcare professionals, engaging in clear, confident, and empathetic discussions about health concerns is pivotal. This approach fosters a welcoming environment where clients can comfortably express their health concerns without fear of judgment. Effective and open communication is key to breaking down the barriers of stigma that often lead individuals to delay seeking the healthcare they need.

Below is a detailed table showcasing specific characteristics and traits associated with various types of social support networks (SSN), including their potential level of support for someone managing a medical diagnosis and associated stigma:

Social Support Network (SSN) Table 1 – Two Example Decks

| Notecard Number | Type of Social Support | Characteristic/Trait | Support Level (1-5) | Description/Context |
|---|---|---|---|---|
| 1 | Family Members | Emotional and practical support, familial bond and obligation. | 4 | Often primary support; may vary based on family dynamics and understanding of medical issues. |
| 2 | Friends | Peer support, shared experiences, social companionship. | 3 | Can provide emotional support and a sense of normalcy, but may lack specialized knowledge. |
| 3 | Healthcare Providers | Professional medical support, guidance, treatment. | 5 | Essential for medical management and advice, though may lack personal connection. |
| 4 | Support Groups | Community understanding, shared experiences, peer advice. | 4 | Offers a sense of belonging and shared understanding, particularly for stigma management. |
| 5 | Mental Health Counselors | Professional emotional and psychological support. | 5 | Crucial for managing mental health aspects of a diagnosis, especially stigma. |

| Notecard Number | Type of Social Support | Characteristic/Trait | Support Level (1-5) | Description/Context |
|---|---|---|---|---|
| 6 | Online Communities | Virtual support, information sharing, accessibility. | 3 | Provides a broad range of perspectives and resources, but may lack personalization. |
| 7 | Faith Leaders/Communities | Spiritual support, moral guidance, community belonging. | 2 | Can offer comfort and a sense of community, though support level varies widely. |
| 8 | Colleagues/Workplace Support | Professional understanding, daily interaction, workplace adjustments. | 2 | Offers a sense of normalcy and routine, but may have limitations in depth of support. |
| 9 | Advocacy Groups | Rights protection, resource provision, community activism. | 3 | Important for addressing systemic issues and providing resources, but less personal. |
| 10 | Educational Institutions | Information, structured support, youth guidance. | 3 | Particularly relevant for younger individuals; offers structured but less personal support. |

This table provides an overview of the potential types and levels of support that various social networks can offer to individuals managing a medical diagnosis and stigma. The scale from 1 to 5 helps to quantify the level of support, with 1 indicating minimal support and 5 indicating very strong support. This information is crucial for understanding and optimizing the support network around someone dealing with health-related challenges.

Below is a detailed table focusing on how the characteristics and traits of various types of social support networks (SSN) are often expressed, along with their corresponding level of support:

| Notecard Number | Type of Social Support | How Characteristics/Traits are Expressed | Support Level (1-5) | Description/Context |
|---|---|---|---|---|
| 1 | Family Members | Through emotional bonding, practical help, presence during medical visits. | 4 | Family often plays a vital role, though the level of support can vary. |
| 2 | Friends | Offering companionship, listening, participating in recreational activities. | 3 | Friends provide a social outlet and emotional support. |
| 3 | Healthcare Providers | Professional advice, medical treatment, follow-up care. | 5 | Essential for medical guidance, though may lack emotional support aspects. |
| 4 | Support Groups | Shared experiences, advice from peers, a sense of community. | 4 | Valuable for feeling understood and receiving peer advice. |
| 5 | Mental Health Counselors | Professional counseling, strategies for coping, emotional support. | 5 | Key for addressing mental health challenges related to diagnosis and stigma. |
| 6 | Online Communities | Sharing experiences online, accessing a wide range of information. | 3 | Provides diverse perspectives and support, but may lack personal interaction. |
| 7 | Faith Leaders/Communities | Spiritual guidance, moral support, community activities. | 2 | Support varies greatly depending on the community and individual belief. |
| 8 | Colleagues/Workplace Support | Workplace adjustments, daily interaction, professional support. | 2 | Offers routine and some support, but often limited in depth. |

| Notecard Number | Type of Social Support | How Characteristics/Traits are Expressed | Support Level (1-5) | Description/Context |
|---|---|---|---|---|
| 9 | Advocacy Groups | Legal advice, fighting for rights, providing specific resources. | 3 | Useful for systemic support and resources, less for personal support. |
| 10 | Educational Institutions | Access to information, structured programs, support from educators. | 3 | Important for younger individuals, offering structured support. |

This table illustrates the various ways in which different social support networks express their support, along with a rating that indicates the typical level of support they provide. The rating scale from 1 to 5 helps to quantify this support, with 1 indicating minimal support and 5 indicating very strong support. This detailed overview is useful for understanding how different types of support manifest and their relative impact on individuals managing medical diagnoses and associated stigma.

## Starting Cohesion's Storytelling Exercises: Building on Foundations to Confront Stigma

As we embark on the storytelling exercise, we're deepening our engagement with the core concepts introduced through Cohesion's innovative training approach. This exercise taps into the collective well of life experiences represented by our cards – Social Support Network (SSN), Age and Diagnostic Setting (ADS), Medical Condition (MC), Population and Target Audience (PT), Stigma by Association (SBA), External Stigma (ES), and Internal Stigma (IS). Each card serves as a narrative fragment, a piece of a larger human story that we will weave together, enhancing our understanding of the complex interplay between individual experiences and societal perceptions.

**Crafting Empathetic Narratives:**

Participants will embark on a creative journey, utilizing the cards to weave narratives that capture the complexities faced by individuals grappling with stigma. This exercise delves deeper than mere recognition of stigma—it's an exploration into the intricacies of the lived experiences of those impacted. We will examine how stigma shapes an individual's ability to seek care and affects the quality of their healthcare encounters. It's important to remember that reactions are not solely based on the words we hear; they are deeply tied to the associations and meanings individuals have internalized regarding those words and their experiences. This understanding is vital in crafting narratives that reflect true understanding and empathy.

**Utilizing the Three Forms of Stigma:**

Each narrative will weave in elements of the three forms of stigma:

1. **Internal Stigma (IS):** Participants will explore the personal struggle where individuals fight against the internalized shame and self-doubt that can erode self-worth and impede the pursuit of care.

2. **External Stigma (ES):** The narratives will reflect on how societal biases and prejudices manifest, affecting individuals' opportunities and creating barriers to healthcare access.

3. **Stigma by Association (SBA):** We'll examine the ripple effect of stigma, considering the impact on friends, family, and communities connected to those living with HIV.

**Empowerment Through Narrative:**

By crafting these stories, participants will gain insight into how individuals mobilize internal and external resources to combat stigma. The process will illustrate not just the challenges but also the resilience and resourcefulness that people can harness.

**Preparing Healthcare Professionals:**

This exercise aims to equip healthcare professionals with a deeper understanding of stigma's multifaceted nature. It will enhance their readiness to encourage the individuals they serve to gather their resources—both within themselves and from the community—to confront stigma head-on as they seek and receive the care they deserve.

**In Summary:**

The storytelling exercise is a crucial step in our journey with Cohesion. It reinforces our earlier learning and propels us into action, preparing us to be not just healthcare providers but also advocates and allies in the fight against stigma. Through this, we will empower those we serve to claim their right to care, support, and dignity.

## Internalized Stigma Storytelling Exercise

**Objective:**
The purpose of this exercise is to utilize a range of card decks to construct detailed characters and their stories, with a focus on the multifaceted impact of internalized stigma. Participants will delve into the various coping mechanisms and healing resources these characters might use. This activity is structured to deepen empathy, confront and dismantle biases, and facilitate the sharing of effective resources for dealing with stigma. Through crafting and sharing these narratives, participants will gain a more nuanced understanding of the complexities surrounding stigma and its effects on individuals.

**Materials Needed:**

- Social Support Network (SSN) Deck

- Age and Diagnostic Setting (ADS) Deck

- Medical Condition (MC) Deck

- Population and Target Audience (PT) Deck

- Stigma by Association (SBA) Card – Use a blank card and create this.

- External Stigma (ES) Card – Use a blank card and create this.
- Internal Stigma (IS) Card – Use a blank card and create this.

**Instructions:**

1. **Shuffling and Selection:**

    - Each participant has one of each deck (SSN, ADS, MC, PT) and each card (SBA, ES, IS).

    - Ask them to shuffle each deck to ensure randomness.

    - Participants then draw the top card from each deck.

2. **Creating a Character and Story:**

    - Using the information on the cards (either from the top or bottom, as they choose), participants will create a character and a backstory.

    - They should consider how the elements from each card interact to form a cohesive narrative.

3. **Developing the Narrative:**

    - Participants will write about their character, focusing on the following aspects:

        - The character's experience with internalized stigma.

        - Coping strategies that the character uses to manage and heal from stigma.

        - Key turning points or moments of realization in the character's journey that contribute to healing and the identification of resources.

4. **Sharing and Discussion:**

    - Once each participant has developed their character and story, they will share it with the group.

    - After each sharing, the group will engage in a discussion about the narrative.

    - The discussion should focus on challenging biases, empathizing with the character's experiences, and sharing potential resources that could aid someone in a similar situation.

5. **Reflection:**

    - After all participants have shared, lead a reflection session.

- Encourage participants to discuss what they learned from the exercise, how it changed their perspective on stigma, and how they can apply these insights in their professional and personal lives.

**Expected Outcome:**

This exercise is crafted to enhance participants' comprehension of the intricate realities individuals face when dealing with medical conditions and the often accompanying stigma. It aims to equip participants with the ability to discern and confront biases, thereby cultivating a more empathetic and knowledgeable stance when engaging with those encountering similar obstacles.

The activity will also serve to refine participants' communication skills, particularly in the nuances of disclosing information, sharing coping mechanisms, and preventing stigma from tainting conversations with clients. It is a critical time to identify and tackle any instances of stigma or bias that emerge within these narratives. Addressing these issues promptly and thoughtfully lays a solid groundwork for all future client interactions.

Additionally, the exercise offers a valuable opportunity for participants to understand and articulate the detrimental effects of stigma. Through active participation in storytelling, individuals can contemplate and articulate the pervasive impact of stigma on a person's well-being. This reflective practice is instrumental in fostering a healthcare environment that is supportive and dignified.

By internalizing these lessons, participants can pass on their enhanced skills, knowledge, and empathetic viewpoints to their clients, who may then extend these benefits to their own support networks, propagating a cycle of understanding and empowerment within the community.

## External Stigma Storytelling Exercise

**Objective:**

The objective of this exercise is to engage with the Social Support Network (SSN), Age and Diagnostic Setting (ADS), Medical Condition (MC), Population and Target Audience (PT), Stigma by Association (SBA), External Stigma (ES), and Internal Stigma (IS) cards and decks to craft comprehensive, empathetic stories. These narratives will focus on individuals navigating various forms of stigma. The aim is to deepen understanding, confront and address any biases, and collaboratively explore supportive resources available for those facing stigma.

**Materials Needed:**

- Decks - SSN, ADS, MC, PT, SBA

- Cards - ES, IS, SBA

**Instructions:**

1. **Shuffling and Selection:** Each participant is given one of each type of card deck. They should shuffle each deck thoroughly to ensure the cards are randomized. Then, they will draw the top card from each deck.

2. **Choosing Card Elements:** Participants can choose to use either the information at the top or bottom of each drawn card to build their narrative. This decision will influence the character and story they create.

3. **Creating a Character and Backstory:** Using the selected card elements, each participant will create a character and develop a backstory. This story should include details about the character's age, diagnosis setting, medical condition, target audience, and experiences with both internal and external stigma.

4. **Exploring External Stigma:** Participants will write about the external stigma their character faces in their life, detailing the societal challenges and prejudices the character encounters.

5. **Coping Strategies:** Narratives should also include the coping strategies the character employs to manage and heal from the stigma. This could include support networks, personal resilience, therapy, etc.

6. **Key Turning Points:** Identify and describe key moments or realizations in the character's journey that could contribute to healing and the discovery of resources.

7. **Sharing and Discussion:** Once everyone has developed their story, each participant will share their narrative with the group. After each sharing, there will be a group discussion focusing on the insights gained, challenging biases, and sharing potential resources that could aid individuals like the character.

8. **Conclusion:** Conclude the exercise by reflecting on the diversity of experiences and challenges faced by individuals dealing with stigma. Emphasize the importance of empathy, understanding, and the need for comprehensive support systems.

**Expected Outcomes:** This exercise is designed to cultivate a profound comprehension of the intricate dynamics involved in medical diagnoses and the associated stigma. Through the creation and exploration of diverse narratives, the activity is structured to augment empathy among participants, confront and reassess any pre-existing biases, and facilitate the exchange of valuable resources and effective strategies. Participants will be better equipped to articulate the nuances of various stigmas and provide insightful guidance, promoting positive change and understanding. This exercise aims to empower healthcare professionals to not only recognize but actively address and alleviate the impacts of stigma in medical contexts. By doing so, they can contribute significantly to improving patient care and fostering a more inclusive and understanding healthcare environment.

## Stigma by Association Storytelling Exercise

**Objective:** The purpose of this exercise is to cultivate empathy and deepen understanding through the development of character narratives. These narratives will encompass diverse elements of stigma, diagnosis, and support. Participants will engage with a range of randomly selected cards from various decks, each card offering a unique piece of a character's life puzzle. Through this creative process, participants will construct a backstory for their character, delving into how they cope with stigma, identifying pivotal moments in their journey, and discovering resources that aid in their resilience and healing. This immersive exercise not only aids in comprehending the multifaceted nature of individuals' experiences with health and stigma but also enhances participants' ability to empathize and connect with the stories of those they may serve or interact with in their professional roles.

**Materials Needed:**

- Social Support Network (SSN) Deck

- Age and Diagnostic Setting (ADS) Deck

- Medical Condition (MC) Deck

- Population and Target Audience (PT) Deck

- Stigma by Association (SBA) Card

- External Stigma (ES) Card

- Internal Stigma (IS) Card

**Instructions:**

1. **Shuffling and Selecting Cards:**

    - Shuffle each of the seven decks separately to randomize the cards.

    - Participants select the top card from each deck.

2. **Character Creation:**

    - Using the information from the selected cards, each participant creates a character. They can choose to use the information from the top or bottom of each card.

    - The character should have a backstory that integrates elements from each card, such as their age, medical condition, social supports, and experiences with different types of stigma.

3. **Narrative Exploration:**

    - Write about how Stigma by Association impacts the character's life.

    - Describe the coping strategies the character employs to manage and heal from stigma.

    - Identify key turning points or moments of realization in the character's journey, focusing on healing and resource identification.

4. **Sharing and Discussion:**

    - Each participant shares their character's story with the group.

    - After each story is shared, engage in a group discussion. Focus on challenging biases, sharing insights, and identifying potential resources that could assist individuals facing similar situations in real life.

5. **Reflective Conclusion:**

- Conclude the exercise with a reflective discussion on the exercise's impact on participants' understanding of stigma, diagnosis, and support networks.

**Outcome:** The goal of this exercise is to enhance participants' comprehension of the intricate realities associated with managing a medical condition while simultaneously confronting stigma. Through the development and exchange of personal narratives, participants are expected to acquire a more nuanced perspective on the layered aspects of stigma. They will explore the pivotal role played by robust support networks, effective coping strategies, and defining moments that are crucial in navigating and surmounting the hurdles posed by their medical and social circumstances. This activity is designed not only to educate but also to foster empathy and a deeper appreciation for the resilience and resourcefulness required in such journeys.

## Group Reflection Session: Implementing a Debriefing for Learning and Insight

**Objective:** The Group Reflection Session is designed to facilitate a debriefing where participants reflect on their learnings from the exercises, particularly focusing on their understanding of stigma, diagnosis, and support systems. The session aims to link these insights to real-world applications, influencing both professional and personal approaches to similar situations.

**Materials Needed:**

- Comfortable seating arrangement for a group discussion.

- Whiteboard or flip chart (optional) for noting key points.

- Handouts for participants to jot down their reflections (optional).

**Session Structure:**

1. **Introduction (5-10 minutes):**

   - Start with a brief introduction, emphasizing the importance of reflection in consolidating learning.

   - Outline the session's objectives and encourage an open, respectful, and non-judgmental atmosphere.

2. **Individual Reflection (10-15 minutes):**

   - Give participants a few minutes to individually reflect on what they learned from the exercises.

   - They can write down their thoughts, focusing on how the activities impacted their understanding of stigma, diagnosis, and support systems.

3. **Facilitated Group Discussion (30-45 minutes):**

   - Open the floor for participants to share their reflections. This can be done in a round-robin format to ensure everyone has a chance to speak.

- Encourage participants to discuss:

    - How the exercises changed or reinforced their views on stigma and diagnosis.

    - Specific insights they gained and how these can be applied in real-life scenarios.

    - The impact of the exercises on their perception of support systems.

- As the facilitator, guide the discussion to keep it on track and ensure that it remains constructive and inclusive.

4. **Linking to Real-World Applications (15-20 minutes):**

- Shift the discussion to how the insights gained can influence professional and personal approaches to handling stigma and supporting individuals with diagnoses.

- Encourage participants to think of specific actions or changes they can implement in their work or personal life.

5. **Noting Key Points and Actionable Steps (10-15 minutes):**

- Use a whiteboard or flip chart to note down key insights and actionable steps discussed during the session.

- Encourage participants to think of at least one action they can commit to as a result of the session.

6. **Conclusion and Feedback (5-10 minutes):**

- Summarize the key points and actions identified during the session.

- Thank participants for their contributions and ask for brief feedback on the session to gauge its effectiveness and areas for improvement.

7. **Follow-Up (Post-Session):**

- Consider sending a follow-up email summarizing the session's key points and reminding participants of their committed actions.

- Optionally, plan a follow-up session to revisit the discussions and actions to assess progress and continued learning.

This Group Reflection Session provides a structured yet flexible format for participants to deeply engage with their learnings, fostering a greater understanding of stigma, diagnosis, and support systems in a real-world context.

**Objective:** The purpose of this workshop is to equip participants with the tools to craft actionable, strategic plans aimed at combatting stigma within their professional environments or broader communities. Drawing upon the knowledge and empathy cultivated in prior sessions, the workshop will guide attendees through the creation of tailored action plans. These plans will not only target the reduction of stigma but also promote inclusivity and understanding, fostering a supportive atmosphere in their respective spheres of influence.

**Materials Needed:**

- Flip charts or whiteboards

- Markers

- Notepads and pens for participants

- Optional: Laptop and projector for presentations

**Duration:** Approximately 2-3 hours

**Workshop Structure:**

1. **Introduction (15 minutes):**

   - Begin with a brief recap of the insights and knowledge gained from the previous exercises on stigma.

   - Introduce the concept of an action plan and its importance in implementing change.

2. **Brainstorming Session (30 minutes):**

   - Divide participants into small groups.

   - Each group brainstorms potential areas within their professional field or community where stigma is prevalent and discusses possible strategies for addressing these issues.

3. **Developing Action Plans (60 minutes):**

   - Guide each group to select one area of focus from their brainstorming session.

   - Groups then develop a detailed action plan for this area. The plan should include specific goals, steps to achieve these goals, required resources, potential challenges, and timelines.

   - Encourage the inclusion of both short-term and long-term strategies.

4. **Presentation of Action Plans (45 minutes):**

   - Each group presents their action plan to the rest of the participants.

   - Encourage constructive feedback and discussion on each plan.

5. **Refinement and Finalization (30 minutes):**

- Based on the feedback received, each group refines their action plan.

- Provide assistance as needed to ensure each plan is practical and achievable.

6. **Conclusion (10 minutes):**

- Summarize the key takeaways from the workshop.

- Discuss the importance of implementing these action plans and the impact they could have.

- Encourage participants to commit to their plans and consider ways to track progress.

**Post-Workshop:**

- Provide participants with a template or digital platform to document and track the progress of their action plans.

- Consider scheduling a follow-up meeting or session to review progress and discuss challenges and successes.

**Notes for Facilitators:**

- Ensure that the workshop is interactive and collaborative.

- Be prepared to offer guidance and support to groups as they develop their action plans.

- Encourage realistic and achievable goal setting.

- Foster an environment of openness where participants feel comfortable sharing ideas and feedback.

This work is made possible by donations to the Crown Legacy, Visibility, and Cultural Catalyst Fund.

We ask that you donate at least $25.00 to this fund and help us with this mission. The link is below and please send a screen capture or email acknowledging your donation with the answers to your assessment.

https://2014givenow.kimbia.com/crownlegacy You may also use the QR code provided below to donate.

**If you are submitting these answers for a certification that is not part of a workshop, please follow these instructions.**

1.    Complete the assessment at the back of this book.

2.    Email your completed assessment to crownhouseone@gmail.com along with your screenshot of a donation.

3.  Your certification will be emailed to you within 2 weeks of reviewing your assessment.

4.  Please put HSA Certification in the subject of your email.

**HSA Certification**

HIV Stigma Abolitionist (HSA) certification designation recognizes healthcare professionals who have completed comprehensive training in culturally competent care practices for individuals affected by HIV. This certification affirms the recipient's commitment to abolishing HIV stigma and creating a more just and equitable society.

**Benefits of HSA Certification:**

1.  **Recognition of Expertise:** Professionals can showcase their specialized training in HIV-related cultural competency, a critical area in healthcare.

2.  **Professional Development:** The certification contributes to ongoing professional education, highlighting a dedication to learning and excellence in patient care.

3.  **Enhanced Trust:** It builds trust with patients, indicating that the professional has a deeper understanding of the social and cultural dimensions of HIV care.

4.  **Career Advancement:** This certification may enhance job prospects, opportunities for advancement, and professional credibility within the healthcare community.

5.  **Continued Education Credits:** The certification could potentially be recognized for continuing education credits, depending on the professional standards and requirements of healthcare institutions or licensing boards.

Welcome to the final step towards earning your HIV Stigma Abolitionist (HSA) certification. This knowledge assessment is designed to evaluate your understanding of key concepts, strategies, and approaches to effectively reduce and address HIV-related stigma. To successfully obtain the HSA certification, you are required to demonstrate a comprehensive grasp of the material by scoring 80% or higher on this assessment. The questions have been carefully crafted to reflect the critical aspects of HIV stigma abolition discussed throughout our program. To earn the HIV Stigma Abolitionist (HSA) certification, participants must achieve a score of 80% or higher.

**1. Which of the following best defines HIV-related stigma?**

     A. General fear about HIV

     B. Discrimination against people living with HIV

     C. Lack of awareness about HIV treatment

     D. The need for more HIV-related research

**2. What is a key factor in reducing HIV stigma in healthcare settings?**

     A. Avoiding discussions about HIV

     B. Providing education about HIV transmission

     C. Offering separate services for HIV patients

     D. Focusing only on medical treatment

**3. How does stigma affect people living with HIV?**

     A. It has no significant effect

     B. It can lead to improved health outcomes

     C. It may discourage individuals from seeking treatment

     D. It only affects mental health

**4. What is an effective strategy for healthcare professionals to combat HIV stigma?**

     A. Avoiding the topic of HIV unless necessary

     B. Using person-first language

     C. Treating HIV patients differently to protect their privacy

     D. Assuming all patients are knowledgeable about HIV

**5. Which of the following is NOT a symptom of internalized HIV stigma?**

     A. Self-isolation

     B. Increased self-esteem

     C. Fear of disclosure

     D. Guilt or shame

**6. What role can healthcare providers play in reducing HIV stigma?**

     A. Only providing medical treatment

     B. Educating patients about HIV transmission and prevention

     C. Avoiding discussions about HIV to prevent discomfort

     D. Focusing solely on physical symptoms

**7. Why is it important to include education about HIV in stigma reduction efforts?**

    A. It is not particularly important

    B. It can lead to increased fear and stigma

    C. Education helps dispel myths and misconceptions

    D. Only medical professionals need HIV education

**8. What is a crucial component of stigma-free communication about HIV?**

    A. Using complex medical terms to explain HIV

    B. Avoiding any discussion of HIV status

    C. Speaking openly and respectfully about HIV

    D. Focusing on the stigma rather than the individual